BENEFIT INCIDENCE

BENEFIT INCIDENCE

PUBLIC HEALTH EXPENDITURES AND INCOME DISTRIBUTION: A CASE STUDY OF COLOMBIA

By

ELKE C. MELDAU

THE CHRISTOPHER PUBLISHING HOUSE
NORTH QUINCY, MASSACHUSETTS

Library of Congress Catalog Card Number 79-90768
ISBN: 0—8158—0389—3

PRINTED IN
THE UNITED STATES OF AMERICA

To my mother

PREFACE

Benefit incidence theory and its applications is a new and important area of research. In many countries, government expenditures represent a significant share of GDP and are expanding rapidly. The actual and potential effect of these expenditures on the distribution of income may be significant. Aware of this, researchers have attempted to quantify the distributional effects of government outlays. These empirical analyses have generated criticism and investigations into the theory and methodology of benefit incidence.

This study brings together various contributions to the labyrinth of Benefit Incidence Theory by a number of economists, including those by: Henry Aaron and Martin McGuire; Shlomo Maital; William Fellner; Kenneth V. Greene, William B. Neenan, and Claudia D. Scott; and Charles E. McLure, Jr. In an Appendix, the study also includes a discussion of the separate but related area of Expenditure Incidence Theory.

The empirical analysis is limited to the area of public health expenditures for several reasons. These include: the distributional implications of public health expenditures in general; and, for practical and conceptual reasons discussed in the text, the importance of limiting the scope of any benefit incidence study in order to be able to consider the distributional impact of possible marginal, rather than overall, changes in public expenditures. The case study was done for Colombia because of its generally good availability of data for a developing country.

Previous investigations into the benefits of health expenditures are discussed and evaluated. The benefit incidence (and, taking into consideration tax incidence, the net fiscal incidence) of public health expenditures in Colombia in 1970 is estimated both on a cost-of-service basis, which is the traditional method for estimating benefit incidence, and on a willingness-to-pay basis, which is shown to be conceptually preferable for the purpose of the analysis.

The author is grateful to Charles T. Stewart, Jr., Professor of Economics, The George Washington University, and to John Eric Fredland, Associate Professor of Economics, U.S. Naval Academy, Annapolis, for their comments and assistance as Director and Co-Director of the research, respectively, when it was being prepared for acceptance as a doctoral dissertation at The George Washington University.

Elke C. Meldau

CONTENTS

Preface 7
1. Theoretical Analysis of Benefit Incidence 15
Introduction
The Theory of Benefit Incidence
Source-of-Income Benefits
Use-of-Income Benefits
Summary
2. Benefits From Public Health Expenditures 57
Introduction
Approaches to the Measurement of Public Health Benefits
Evaluation of Existing Methods and Concepts
Mishan's Theoretical Approach to the Evaluation of Human Life
Measurement and Imputation of Public Health Benefits in Previous Fiscal Incidence Studies
Survey of Previous Studies
Evaluation of Previous Studies
Summary
3. The Public Health Sector in Colombia 92
Introduction
Historical Evolution of Health Policy
Health Systems in Colombia
Initiatives Taken During the 1960's
The Ministry of Public Health
Introduction
Health Protection and Promotion
Health Recuperation
The Colombian Social Security Institute
Introduction
Insurance Programs and Administration
Health Services
Summary

4. The Redistributive Impact of Public Health Expenditures in Colombia on the Distribution of Income 118
Introduction
The Ministry of Public Health
The Distribution of Income Among Colombian Households, 1970
The Distribution of National Taxes by Income Groups, 1970
The Distribution of Benefits Generated by Health Expenditures of the Ministry of Public Health by Income Class, 1970
The Net Fiscal Incidence of Health Expenditures of the Ministry of Public Health by Income Class, 1970
The Colombian Social Security Institute
The Distribution of Income Among Colombian Workers Insured by ICSS, 1970
The Distribution of Social Security Contributions by Income Class, 1970
The Distribution of Benefits Generated by Health Expenditures of the Colombian Social Security Institute by Income Class, 1970
Net Fiscal Incidence of Health Expenditures of the Colombian Social Security Institute by Income Class, 1970
Summary
5. Summary and Conclusions 179
General Introduction
Summary of Empirical Results
The Future of Health Policy in Colombia
Financing a Higher Level of Public Health Expenditures
Conceptual and Statistical Limitations of the Analysis
General Conclusion
Appendix 1 The Theory of Expenditure Incidence 193
Appendix 2 The Level and Pattern of Private Expenditures on Health Care, 1970 201
Selected Bibliography 205
Index 215

LIST OF ILLUSTRATIONS

FIGURES

1. Effects of government expenditures on the welfare of individuals 20
2. Exposition of the Aaron and McGuire Method for measuring the income value of a pure public good to a given individual 30
3. Exposition of the Aaron and McGuire Method for imputing the income value of a pure public good to two given individuals 31
4. Illustration of the two conditions which must be fulfilled for total government expenditures to equal total marginal benefits received by individuals: (1) optimal provision of public services and (2) constant marginal cost of provision 42
5. Model of an optimal social welfare criterion imposed by an omniscient and benevolent dictator 43
6. Individualistic collective decision-making model: a purely democratic decision-making process is assumed in which individuals differ and the output level is controlled by the median or representative voter 45
7. Mishan's theoretical approach to the evaluation of human life: analysis of risks associated with projects which increase or reduce the risk of death, injury or disease 62
8. Colombia: Lorenz Curves for 1970 123
9. Expenditure Incidence: Price Effects and Employment Effects 197
10. Expenditure Incidence: Determinants of the Effects of Government Expenditures on Relative Prices 198

TABLES

1. Distribution of use-of-income benefits under three different utility assumptions 35
2. Bases employed by Gillespie to allocate expenditures on public health, hospital care, and sanitation by income class 70
3. Ministry of Public Health: total expenditures by function, 1970 98
4. Ministry of Public Health: current and investment expenditures by function, 1970 99
5. Colombian Social Security Institute: health, disability, and retirement insurance 105
6. Colombian Social Security Institute: expenditures under insurance programs, 1970 111
7. Estimated distribution of income among urban households, 1970 121
8. Estimated distribution of income among rural households, 1970 122
9. Estimated distribution of income among Colombian households, 1970 125
10. Colombia: total national tax collections by type of tax, 1970 127
11. Allocation of national taxes among households 133
12. Effective rates of national taxation, all households 134
13. Ministry of Public Health: distribution of health service benefits by income class—cost-of-service basis 136
14. Ministry of Public Health: distribution of health service benefits by income class—willingness-to-pay basis 138
15. Ministry of Public Health: net fiscal residuals by income class —benefits estimated on a cost-of-service basis 142
16. Ministry of Public Health: net fiscal residuals by income class—benefits estimated on a willingness-to-pay basis 143
17. Colombian Social Security Institute: revenues for general health and maternity services, 1970 145
18. Colombian Social Security Institute: estimated distribution of income among workers insured by ICSS, 1970 147
19. Colombian Social Security Institute: number of insured workers by economic activity, 1970 148
20. Ministerio del Trabajo y Seguridad Social, Instituto Colombiano de Seguros Sociales: categorias de salarios y aportes vigentes desde el 1° de septiembre de 1965—decreto N° 1825 de 1965 (cajas seccionales de Antioquia y Valle del Cauca y oficina local de Santa Marta) 152

21. Ministerio del Trabajo y Seguridad Social, Instituto Colombiano de Seguros Sociales: categorias de salarios y aportes vigentes desde el 1º de septiembre de 1965—decreto Nº 1825 de 1965 (cajas seccionales de Cundinamarca y Quindio y officinas locales (excepto Santa Marta) 153
22. Colombian Social Security Institute: allocation of social security contributions and other sources of revenue among affiliated workers by income class, 1970 155
23. Colombian Social Security Institute: effective rates of social security taxation and other taxes levied in order to finance health services, through the Colombian Social Security Institute, 1970 156
24. Colombian Social Security Institute: distribution of health service benefits by income class, 1970 158
25. Colombian Social Security Institute: number of days and cases of incapacity by income class, 1970 160
26. Colombian Social Security Institute: number of cases and days of incapacity by groups of causes and income bracket, 1970 161
27. Colombian Social Security Institute: number of cases and days of incapacity by groups of causes and income bracket, 1970 (percentage distribution) 162
28. Colombian Social Security Institute: number of cases and days of incapacity with subsidies paid by age groups, 1970 164
29. Colombian Social Security Institute: number of cases and days of incapacity by economic sector, 1970 165
30. Colombian Social Security Institute: number of cases and days of incapacity by economic sector, 1970 166
31. Colombian Social Security Institute: net fiscal residuals—benefits estimated on a cost-of-service basis and on a willingness-to-pay basis 168
32. Private health expenditure patterns in urban areas by income class, 1970 202
33. Households purchasing selected health services in urban areas by income class, 1970 203

Chapter 1

THEORETICAL ANALYSIS OF BENEFIT INCIDENCE

Introduction

Real gross national product of many developing countries increased at unprecedented rates over the past decade.[1] However, relatively little of this growth filtered down to the poorest segments of the population. Raising the income of the poor is included among the development goals of most countries, but very few have undertaken significant measures to achieve this objective. Countries need to base the allocation of public resources for development purposes not only on the contribution a particular project could make to total output but also on the distribution of benefits to be expected. Concern with this problem is only beginning to be reflected in the operations of external lending agencies such as, for example, the World Bank. Economic performance is beginning to be evaluated on the basis of social indicators, and the type of projects eligible for financing is also changing.

Due to the relative importance of government in most developing countries, it appears *a priori* that government could play a decisive role in changing the distribution of income. Recognition of this possibility is not new, and a considerable number of studies have examined the distributional impact of government budgetary policies focusing, however, almost exclusively on tax incidence. A new area of research opened up in recent years in which the distributional effects of public expenditures are examined, although such studies are still scarce, particularly for developing countries. Economists are realizing that the distributive role of the tax system is limited and that remedies for poverty must come through the expenditure side of the budget. The existence of a relatively progressive income tax may be one of the causes of the low tax burden in some countries, as it may persuade the average citizen that his tax burden is not light. Vito Tanzi, in criticizing the excessive emphasis upon equity in the Fiscal Reform for Colombia prepared several years ago by the Musgrave Commission,[2] the major part of which was adopted during the latter months of 1974, made the following suggestions: ". . . I wonder whether a better, or one could say a more cynically pragmatic strategy would not have been to try to increase the tax ratio by raising the taxes which are least 'felt' by the tax payer and copying this with a substantial increase in those expenditures which help the lower classes . . . ignore the equity aspect of taxation but raise as much as you can and then worry about equity when you use the revenues. It may offend the purist, but in some cases it is the only feasible solution."[3] Others have pointed out that the standard of living of the poor is not improved by not taxing them. It is through direct public expenditures on such services as housing, education, and health, or by instituting employment-creating policies or even by direct income transfers that the standard of living of the poor can be improved.[4] Furthermore, the distributional impact of government expenditures may be significant, whether or not they are intended to redistribute incomes, as these generally amount to a large proportion of GDP.

Systematic inquiries into the incidence of current patterns of public expenditures by size classes of income are being undertaken in order to determine where these resources really go and which income groups benefit most. Governments may use these studies as a basis for constructing development programs which will improve the distribution of services provided by the public sector. In urging governments to initiate studies of benefit incidence, the president of the World Bank, Robert S. McNamara, stated at the IBRD/IMF Annual Meeting in 1972: "Too often these expenditures—on health, on transport, on water supply, on education, and on many other sectors—end by benefiting the already privileged far more than the mass of the disadvantaged. This, in part, is because these services are more concentrated in the urban areas and better neighborhoods."[5]

This study is concerned primarily with allocating the benefits from government expenditures by income class, focusing the empirical analysis on the incidence of public health expenditures in Colombia. The objective is to determine whether public expenditures on health programs in Colombia improve the distribution of income. A section will also be devoted to tax incidence in Colombia in order to estimate the net fiscal incidence of public health expenditures. (Total taxes paid will be reduced to the level of public health expenditures and allocated among taxpayers according to the estimated distribution of tax burdens.) In the light of these estimates, such questions will be addressed as: what would be the best way to use public health expenditures to redistribute income, who will bear the burden of additional expenditures on public health, and how should the costs be shared between the taxpayers and beneficiaries.

The revenue and expenditure aspects of governmental activity need to be combined in order to estimate the entire redistributional impact or net fiscal incidence of a public service provided through the budget. To divert resources from the private to the public sector, governments may use various methods, each with a different effect on an individual's income position relative to others. His relative income position is altered by the taxes he pays and by the value of the benefits he receives from public services. This change in his relative income position due to the tax and expenditure policies of the public sector is known as the net fiscal incidence. Net fiscal incidence, therefore, concerns measurement of the change in real income of various groups due to the tax and expenditure activities of the government.

The problem may be formulated as follows:

$$\Delta Y = Y_1 + G_1 - Y_0$$

where ΔY represents the change in real income of any household, Y_0 private and total real income prior to the existence of government, and Y_1 and G_1 measure private real income and the real income-equivalent of public services consumed by the household, respectively, given the existence of government.[6]

In the following sections of this chapter, the theory of benefit incidence will be discussed. Studies concerned with the benefits of public health expenditures, their measurement and imputation by income class, will be surveyed and evaluated in Chapter 2. The public health sector in Colombia will be discussed in Chapter 3, particularly the expenditures in fiscal 1970 of the Ministry of Public Health and health expenditures of the Colombian Social Security Institute during the same year. In Chapter 4, the estimates of tax incidence, benefit incidence, and net fiscal incidence are presented under various assumptions. Finally, in Chapter 5, a number of relevant theoretical, empirical, and policy issues will be discussed.

Analysis of how government expenditures affect the distribution of income has been referred to as *expenditure incidence*, and this needs to be distinguished from *benefit incidence*, which is concerned with the problem of determining who benefits from these expenditures.[7] This study is concerned with the latter. However, there also is a discussion of the theory of expenditure incidence in Appendix 1.

The Theory of Benefit Incidence

The theory of public finance has devoted considerable attention to the welfare gains generated by government expenditures, but attempts to allocate these gains across income classes employing the methodology developed for tax incidence analysis are, as mentioned earlier, relatively recent. Allocating the benefits of public services involves difficult theoretical and empirical questions. For example, the direct recipients of these services may not be the only beneficiaries. Upper income groups financing services intended to benefit the poor are also thought to benefit, and this may be supported both theoretically and empirically. Interdependent utility functions and the existence of externalities, as they are usually defined, are the basis for the theoretical argument. Empirical evidence is derived from the "willingness-to-pay" for these expenditures by upper income groups. If new policies are to be formulated to correct inequities, empirical measures of the benefits from public services are needed and one of the main objectives of this study is to explore the usefulness of alternative measures of these benefits. The development of the individualistic,[8] in contrast to the collectivistic,[9] approach to economic analysis has had a significant bearing upon the manner in which it is thought that benefit incidence should be measured. Individuals satisfy certain wants by purchasing goods and services in the market and other wants collectively through the provision of public services. The state, according to the individualistic approach, exists solely for the purpose of fulfilling the wants of its individual members and its decisions are the collective decisions of its members rather than those of a separate decision-making unit. It is the individual, therefore, who is regarded as the recipient of benefits provided by government expenditures.

Public expenditure analysis and economic theory have been formally integrated in discussions relating the level of public output to individual utility maximization, but economists are still working toward a generally acceptable technique for evaluating the benefits from government expenditures that might be compared to the measurement of private goods and services in the national accounts. Although notable advances have been made in identifying, measuring, and imputing the benefits generated by the provision of public services, the conceptual and empirical problems involved in this analysis will probably remain the subject of research for many years before a methodology comparable to that employed in tax incidence analysis becomes generally accepted.

Government expenditures affect the welfare of an individual

through (1) the effects of the expenditures themselves upon his "sources of income" and (2) the consumption satisfaction that he derives from the "use of income" to provide public services. Various studies have identified what are regarded as the main effects of government expenditures upon the welfare of individuals and suggested procedures for quantifying them.[10] These effects are summarized in Figure 1, which will provide a framework for the discussion below.

Source-of-income Benefits

Government expenditures are either money transfers to individuals or exhaustive expenditures, both of which generate increased income or source-of-income benefits for individuals. Money transfers, such as welfare payments to the poor, increase the personal income of recipients directly. Exhaustive expenditures generate increased income through in-kind transfers, such as services provided gratis to certain groups, and through general equilibrium adjustments resulting from the purchase of factors of production. (see Figure 1.) The following discussion is concerned with the appropriate procedures for estimating each of these three source-of-income benefits.

Money transfers

As a measure of the direct (source-of-income) benefits or welfare gain, benefit incidence studies generally have taken the full value of money transfers and allocated them to recipients. Money transfers are thus treated as negative personal taxes and analyzed using the methodology developed for tax incidence analysis.

Theoretically, the net gain to recipients should be determined by adding the value of increased leisure time to the value of the money transfer and then subtracting the income which would have been earned if the transfer had not been made. Owing to the practical problems in estimating these adjustments, however, the full value of cash transfers has generally served as a measure of (source-of-income) benefits generated.[11]

In-kind transfers

Government expenditures generate source-of-income benefits when they are explicitly used to redistribute income by providing public services free of charge to certain groups. These services cannot be regarded as generating use-of-income benefits for the same groups.

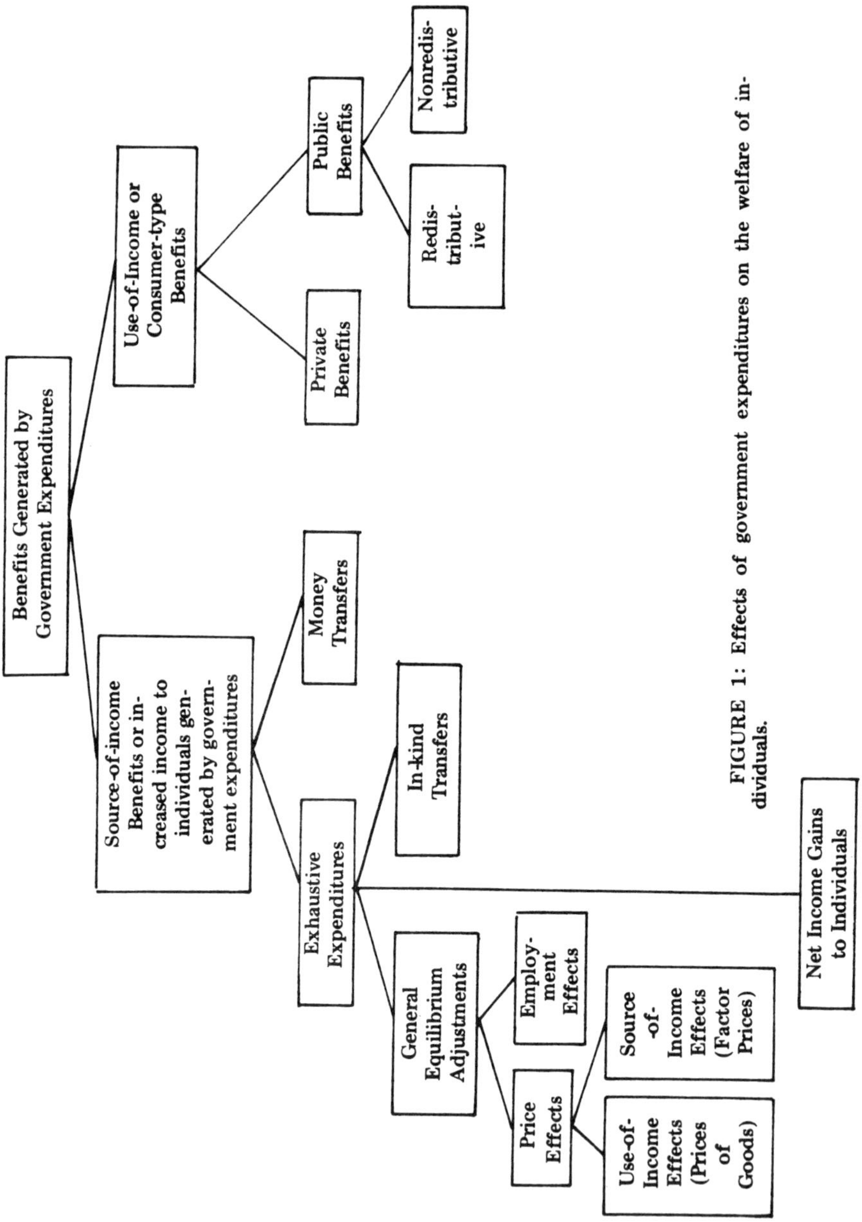

FIGURE 1: Effects of government expenditures on the welfare of individuals.

They do, however, generate use-of-income benefits for those who are willing and able to finance them with their taxes, that is, those who have an effective demand for them.

The welfare gain to recipients is usually measured as the money cost of providing the in-kind transfers, but the value of in-kind transfers to the recipients may be less than their cost. Consumption choices may be constrained by providing in-kind rather than money transfers. Some authors have suggested using specific benefit weights to adjust in-kind benefits to money equivalents.[12] A benefit weight is the ratio of the value placed upon these benefits by the recipient to the market value of the transfer. This ratio should normally range from zero to one. However, many forms of in-kind transfers may be available to low-income recipients, as, for example, education, subsidized housing, health services, agricultural extension services, and food subsidies, thereby reducing the constraints on consumption and increasing the likelihood that the benefit weight may be close to one. This consideration and the lack of empirical research necessary to operationalize this adjustment have resulted in the continued use of the cost of providing in-kind transfers as a measure of benefits.

Factor payments

By purchasing factors of production, a government may initiate general equilibrium adjustments which can generate increased income for individuals. Thorough examination of these adjustments requires the use of an adequately structured general equilibrium model, such as that constructed by McLure.[13] In Appendix 1, some of the theoretical contributions to the analysis of these general equilibrium adjustments are mentioned. A discussion of the significance of *expenditure incidence* analysis, or the analysis of how government expenditures affect the distribution of income; a summary of the three approaches which may be employed in expenditure incidence analysis: (1) *balanced-budget* incidence, (2) *differential* expenditure incidence, and (3) *specific* expenditure incidence; and a summary of the determinants of expenditure incidence, also are included in Appendix 1.

In order to measure the net income gains generated by factor payments, salary payments made to public employees need to be compared to what could have been obtained in the absence of government expenditures. In the national accounts, these appear as personal income, but this clearly overstates the net gain to recipients from these expenditures.

Measurement of the net gain to salary earners employed by the government depends upon whether there is full or less than full employment. In the case of *full employment*, all public employees could have obtained employment elsewhere, but not at a higher, and perhaps at a lower, salary. A public employee's net income gain or loss is therefore the difference between his government-paid wage and the wage he could have received if the government had not paid his wage. Under full employment, increased real income to one individual necessarily means reduced real income for another. Comprehensive analysis of source-of-income benefits, for this reason, should include the losses and the gains, and these must be equal across all households in the case of full employment. In the case of *less than full employment*, the net benefits to a public employee and to society are greater, since some of these employees might have been unemployed in the absence of the government outlay. Under less than full employment, measurement of a public employee's net gain would require weighting the wage he might expect to receive elsewhere by the probability of his being unemployed in the absence of the government expenditure. The difference between his actual wage and his expected wage, weighted in this way, may be called his source-of-income benefit. The "net benefits" to society, furthermore, are greater than zero but less than total government expenditures on wages, unless the extreme case of total unemployment is assumed.[14]

Use-of-Income Benefits

Individuals obtain consumer-type or use-of-income benefits from purchasing public services, as they obtain consumer satisfaction from purchasing privately provided commodities. The individual, in the final analysis, is the recipient of benefits generated by public services whether these involve specific services to a limited group of identifiable recipients, specific services providing both benefits to direct recipients and external benefits to others, or pure public goods consumed in equal amounts by all members of society. His utility function is comprised of public and private goods and the quantity of each provided should be related to utility.[15] The objective of the following analysis is to place the evaluation of public services on the same basis as the evaluation of private services. As consumer surpluses inherent in the consumption of private goods are ignored in national accounting, the consumer surplus provided by inframarginal units of public services are ignored here.

In the private sector, the socially optimal output or allocation of resources to a product or service is defined as the level at which marginal cost equals the price that consumers are willing to pay for the marginal unit, and this is a particular case of the more general definition of optimal output for public goods. The socially optimal level of output of a public good is defined as the quantity at which the sum of the marginal evaluations, or marginal rates of substitution, of all households equals the marginal cost of the public good. The tax price for any household need not equal its marginal rate of substitution, but the sum of the tax payments must equal the sum of the marginal evaluations and this must equal the marginal cost of the public good at the amount supplied. If the condition for social optimality is met, the value of that output, evaluated at the margin, will only equal total costs if the marginal cost of providing the service is constant. Marginal evaluations will be positive for those receiving direct or indirect use-of-income benefits.

The efficiency question, or the relationship between total government outlays and the total money value of use-of-income benefits, is discussed in a subsequent section of this chapter.

Previous benefit incidence studies generally classify public expenditures as either providing benefits to specific groups or as pure public goods, consumed in equal amounts by all members of society. While the benefits of some public services may be limited to direct beneficiaries, most public services involve consumption externalities to other individuals.[16] For example, some individuals enjoy protection from disease because others have been vaccinated, and society as a whole enjoys cultural benefits generated by educational expenditures. These external "spillover benefits" need to be distinguished from other external benefits which arise when money or in-kind transfers are given to certain groups without receiving any return value. Such transfers not only generate welfare or source-of-income benefits to recipients who have not incurred any tax liability *qua* recipients but also "taxpayer benefits" or "public redistributive benefits," as various authors have labelled them.[17]

Classification of use-of-income benefits

Three consumer-type or use-of-income benefits are generated by publicly provided services: (1) private benefits, (2) public nonredistributive benefits, and (3) public redistributive benefits. Each of these would serve as a basis for assigning tax liability under a benefit tax regime.

Private benefits

Private use-of-income benefits are received directly by limited, identifiable groups. Although there may be close market substitutes, the services which generate such benefits are provided publicly.

Public nonredistributive benefits

Public nonredistributive benefits concern the benefits that are generated by pure public goods, or services that are characterized by non-exclusion and non-rivalry in consumption, such as national defense. They also are associated with the public aspects of specific goods. When specific expenditures provide benefits for direct recipients, spillover or external benefits may accrue to other individuals. Since some public services, such as education, provide both private benefits to identifiable recipients and public nonredistributive benefits to society as a whole, total use-of-income benefits need to be distributed between these categories.

Public redistributive benefits

Public redistributive benefits are taxpayer benefits to those who are willing and able to pay for the redistributive source-of-income benefits provided by money and in-kind transfers to low income groups.

The willingness of individuals to pay for redistributive services may be attributed to (1) philanthropy or genuine altruism,[18] (2) recripocal exchange or what appears to be philanthropy but is really given on an implicit *quid pro quo* basis, [19] e.g. social security and unemployment compensation programs (3) the "Kantian Motive,"[20] or the satisfaction derived from the "act" of doing good; whereas genuine altruism is motivated by the result which it brings about, in this case, the individual is motivated by the utility he derives from the act of performing a good deed, rather than a genuine concern with the result; (4) to maintain the dominant positions of the economically and politically privileged by controlling or "buying-off" the lower classes.[21] This "willingness-to-pay" for redistributive programs appears to be greater when other individuals in relatively the same economic position also contribute similar amounts;[22] when the contribution is neither expected to threaten his relative position in the rank order of income,[23] nor significantly change the rank order of income for society,[24] and if psychological attitudes toward low income groups based upon degree and quality of contact encourage such support,[25] and appears to rise with the individual's absolute level of income.

Hochman and Rodgers argue that the Pareto criterion may require that transfers be made from higher to lower income groups because "... the utility of individuals with higher incomes depends upon and is positively related to the incomes of persons lower in the distributive scale ...."[26] Individuals may be willing to pay for redistributive programs because they derive utility or satisfaction from the income transfer for the four reasons mentioned above, all of which may be included under the Pareto criterion.

The rationale for the Hochman and Rodgers analysis is based upon their interpretation of the misleading reasoning implied in the neoclassical approach to public finance, represented by Richard A. Musgrave. The neoclassical approach separates the functions of government and the budget process into three parts: the allocation branch, the distribution branch, and the stabilization branch. This framework provides the basis for constructing a normative theory of the budget based on consumer sovereignty. Under this normative theory, the Pareto criterion is only applied to allocative activities and only to the provision of public goods that are not merit wants. The authors consider this reasoning misleading, as it appears to indicate that consumer sovereignty and redistribution and stabilization cannot be consistent and that individuals who finance redistribution do not enjoy benefits therefrom, only loss. They argue that if this were accepted, redistribution by government could only be interpreted as "legalized Robin Hood activity" and privately financed redistribution would appear to suggest that individuals are irrational.[27] They state that while redistribution may be partially attributable to the political power of recipients, it may also reflect benefits to taxpayers. Their analysis is based on the view that the same methodology and the same criterion—efficiency or Pareto optimality—may be applied to both allocation and redistribution. Using a two-person case, the analysis is based upon the following assumptions:[28]

(a) Both individuals have marginal utilities of income for own consumption greater than zero ($\partial u/\partial y > 0$);

(b) All transfers are required to be Pareto optimal, that is they must not injure or reduce the welfare of either individual;

(c) All transfers flow from the higher income individual to the lower income individual. Given these assumptions, they ask "... under what assumptions about utility interdependence would the actual fiscal structure be Pareto optimal?"[29]

Employing Gillespie's estimates of the net incidence of taxes and expenditures in the U.S. in 1960, they derive fiscal residuals in absolute terms for average individuals in each income bracket. By assuming that these actual fiscal residuals (defined as the benefits of expenditures and transfers received less taxes paid) were Pareto optimal, that is, that they reflect the redistribution of income necessary to internalize interdependence among individual utility functions, they infer values for the transfer-elasticities or the willingness of individuals at upper and middle income levels to transfer income to lower income individuals. They conclude that ". . . since the middle income groups . . . seem, more or less, to break even in the fiscal process, it would appear that utility interdependence increases in significance as income increases and becomes really significant only when income reaches a level of $10,000 or more."[30]

Several authors have commented upon the Hochman and Rodgers paper.[31] Mishan, in criticizing the paper, pointed out that efficiency-derived distributions may be undesirable.[32] He states that first, the pursuit of allocative efficiency may involve only a "potential," rather than an actual, Pareto improvement. (If gains exceed losses, or the gainers can compensate the losers, the criterion for a potential Pareto improvement is met, as in cost-benefit analysis.) Furthermore, when externalities are introduced into the allocative problem, the existence of both malevolence, or perhaps envy, and benevolence must be recognized. He states that if Pareto efficiency required the poor, on balance, to transfer income to the rich due to envy and malevolence as they exist in the real world, those favoring efficiency distributions might either demur or restate their positions. They might in that case support efficiency distributions only under the condition that they reduce income inequality. Mishan points out that policies then would rest on another principle, a principle presumably related to equity. He asserts that the welfare economist's propositions and recommendations need to be based on the ethics of society rather than on utility.[33]

Musgrave regards the Hochman and Rodgers analysis as ". . . a helpful and down-to-earth addition to other recent efforts in this direction. Now that the case has been made, it is indeed difficult to see why this aspect had so long been neglected."[34] However, Musgrave argues that only part of the distribution issue is resolved by the Hochman and Rodgers analysis. He states that through the political process the initial distribution of income, determined by such factors as inheritance, education, and market structures, may be changed. He refers to such changes as "primary redistribution" and regards them as a matter of taking rather than voluntary giving. While Musgrave argues that primary redistribution is a function of the balance of power between income classes and the social structure, "secondary redistribution" is a function of both the initial distribution of income and a person's rate of substitution between the satisfaction derived from giving income and retaining it. Musgrave states that he had primary redistribution in mind when he distinguished between the allocation and distribution branches of government in his own writings and that by allowing for Pareto optimal or secondary redistribution, part of the distribution issue is transferred to the allocation branch. He criticizes Hochman and Rodgers for classifying both categories of redistribution as secondary redistribution.

In their reply to Musgrave's criticism, Hochman and Rodgers state that primary redistribution is not a matter of taking but rather a matter of social contract.[35] They argue that through the constitutional choice process, a society's common and individual rights to human and other resources are established, and that a society produced by a consensus of free individuals has Pareto optimal characteristics, including distributional characteristics. They also argue that it would be unrealistic to regard all redistribution as Pareto optimal, and that they had not intended to give that impression in the paper.

Greene, Neenan, and Scott criticize two of the implicit assumptions underlying the results obtained by Hochman and Rodgers, namely that (1) all government expenditures may be regarded as a means of achieving redistribution, and that (2) expenditures by society as a whole only generate use-of-income consumer benefits, which were allocated in proportion to income.[36] They stress the need to distinguish between programs which are intended to achieve redistribution goals and those which are not. Making this distinction is essential in order to be able to further distinguish between benefits which give rise to tax liability in a benefit-tax system, or use-of-income benefits, and benefits which do not give rise to tax liability, or source-of-income benefits. In terms of the framework illustrated in Figure 1, for example, Hochman and Rodgers fail to acknowledge the existence of public redistributive benefits, or the receipt of use-of-income benefits by taxpayers who finance redistributive programs.

Imputation of Use-of-Income Benefits by Income Class

In this section, the theoretical and empirical contributions to the development of a method for imputing use-of-income benefits by income class are discussed. In particular, it includes a discussion of: (1) the method for measuring and imputing the benefits of pure public goods developed by Aaron and McGuire; (2) the functional relationship between marginal utility and income and efforts to measure it in recent years; and (3) the willingness-to-pay approach for imputing use-of-income benefits to income classes.

The Aaron-McGuire Theorem

Aaron and McGuire have developed an elegant, theoretically founded method for measuring and imputing the benefits from pure public goods to income classes.[37] The method is based upon the proposition, attributable to Mazzola, that each individual's share of the cost of public goods, namely his taxes, should be equal to the marginal utility that these goods provide him.[38] Lindahl later combined Mazzola's basic idea with a theory of collective choice, which became the foundation of the benefit theory of taxation.[39] Aaron and McGuire have clarified and extended the Lindahl model. Employing the following assumptions: (1) "Each household's marginal rate of substitution between public goods and other goods is known, or assumed." (2) "The total and marginal cost of public and specific goods is known for all relevant outputs of these goods." (3) "All utility functions are identical." (4) "All of each public good enters every household's utility function." (5) "All households in each income bracket can be represented by the average income level and expenditure mix in that bracket." (6) "The marginal cost of public goods equals the average cost at the amount supplied." (7) "The actual output of public and specific goods is allocatively efficient, so that marginal cost equals the sum of marginal rates of substitution (MC = Σ MRS). (8) "The utilities of public goods and of other goods are independent.", they show that ". . . *to each household should be imputed a fraction of the total value of the public good, proportional to the reciprocal of its marginal utility of private good expenditure.*"[40] (Emphasis mine.) This is known as the Aaron-McGuire Theorem.

The Aaron and McGuire method and the reasoning underlying it are illustrated below, using a simplified diagram and exposition developed by Maital.[41] Assume that indifference maps for public goods and private goods, regarding the latter as synonymous with disposable income, are known for all individuals. Assume also that the indifference curves for some individual A are represented in Figure 2, that individual A consumes OG units of pure public goods, the same amount as all other individuals in society, and that his gross income (before tax), taxes (less transfers), and disposable income are OD, AD, and OA, respectively. Point C lies on some indifference curve, U_A, in A's preference map and its coordinates are OA and OG. The value to individual A of OG units of public goods may be determined by extending a tangent to indifference curve U_A at point C, intersecting the vertical axis at A'. The slope of A'C measures the marginal rate of substitution or the subjective value to A of one unit of public goods in terms of income. The income value of OG to individual A is therefore AA'. It indicates that "*. . . the income value to each household of the public good equals the product of MRS^i and the amount of public good.*"[42] (Emphasis, mine.) The equality between the income value of a public good and the product of quantity times MRS is exactly analogous to the equality between the income value of a private good and the product of quantity times MRS, which is equated to price when utility is maximized. AA' represents the amount of taxes that individual A would be willing to pay for OG units of public goods under a benefit tax system if he revealed his preferences. This is the Lindahl solution; if taxes were levied according to the benefit principle, this would be A's share. Taxes levied for redistribution purposes alone are represented therefore by DA'.

While AA' represents the income value to A of OG units of public goods, it does not measure the full benefits to A from provision of the public good. Aaron and McGuire employ the term "value" in its neo-classical sense of exchange value, that is, marginal utility times quantity. Exchange value excludes infra-marginal utility gains or consumer surplus which would be included in a measure of "value in use."[43]

In order to illustrate the Aaron and McGuire method for imputing the value of a pure public good to income classes, the following discussion includes two individuals.[44] Assume that there are two individuals, A and B, with identical indifference maps which may be represented by an additively separable utility function for public and private goods. Assume that both individuals consume the same quantity of a public good, OG units, but B's income is higher than A's. Because their incomes differ, the evaluation of the Gth unit differs for each individual. In Figure 3, the value of OG units to A is AA', calculated by multiplying A's marginal rate of substitution (MRS) between public and private goods, namely the slope of the indifference curve at C_A, by OG units. The value of OG units to B is equal to BB' in Figure 3, determined in the same way. In notational form, this procedure may be illustrated as follows:

(1) $AA' = (\text{slope } A'C_A).\ OG.$
(2) $BB' = (\text{slope } B'C_B).\ OG.$

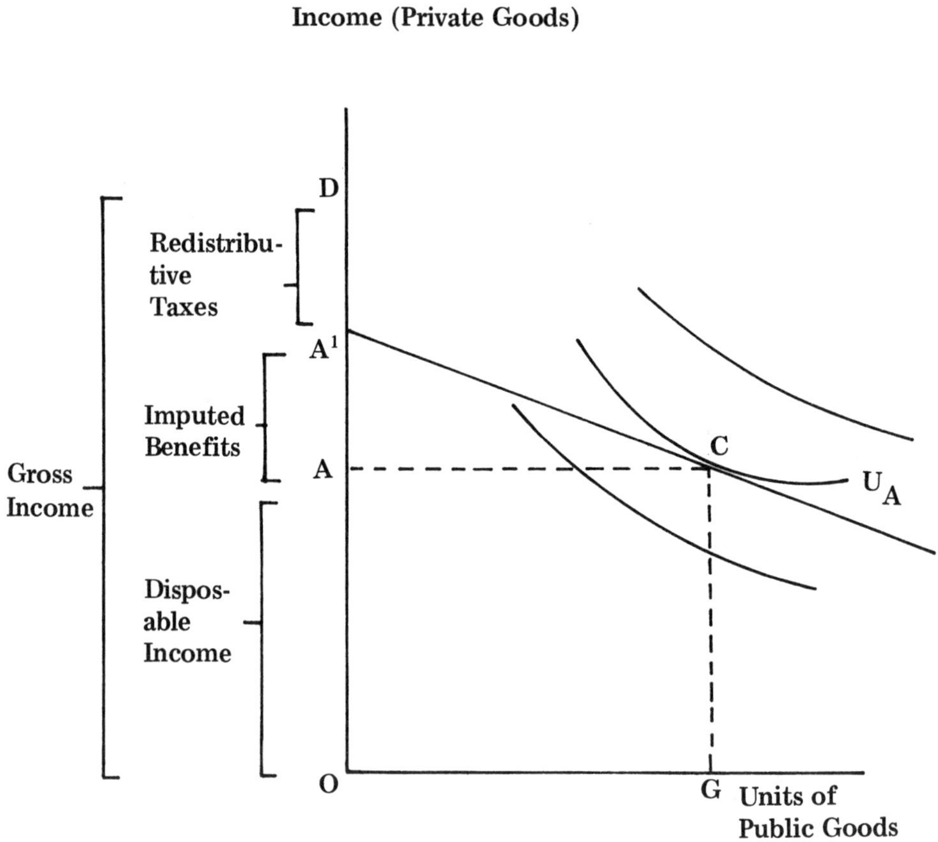

FIGURE 2: Exposition of the Aaron and McGuire Method for measuring the income value of a pure public good to a given individual.

Source: Shlomo Maital, "Public Goods and Income Distribution: Some further Results," p. 563.

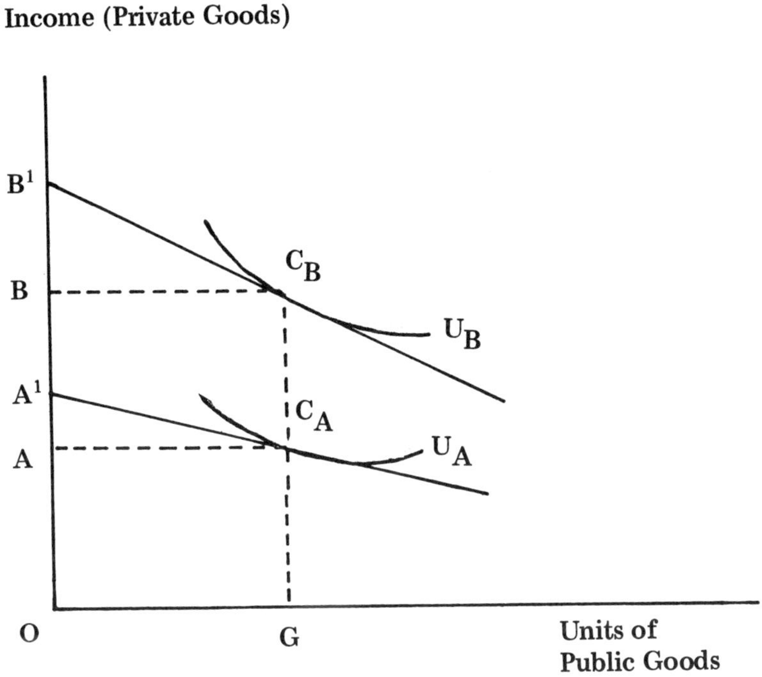

FIGURE 3: Exposition of the Aaron and McGuire Method for imputing the income value of a pure public good to two given individuals.

Source: Greene, Neenan, and Scott, *Fiscal Interactions in a Metropolitan Area*, p. 24.

Dividing (2) by (1),

(3) $BB'/AA' = \text{slope } B'C_B/\text{slope } A'C_A$.

By definition,

$$(4)\ \text{slope } B'C_B = \frac{(\text{marginal utility of OG})_B}{(\text{marginal utility of income})_B}$$

and

$$(5)\ \text{slope } A'C_A = \frac{(\text{marginal utility of OG})_A}{(\text{marginal utility of income})_A}$$

Substituting (4) and (5) into (3),

$$(6)\ \frac{BB'}{AA'} = \frac{(\text{marginal utility of OG})_B}{(\text{marginal utility of income})_B} \Big/ \frac{(\text{marginal utility of OG})_A}{(\text{marginal utility of income})_A}$$

Assuming identical, separable utility functions for public and private goods, the marginal utility of OG units of public goods is equal for both individuals:

(7) $(\text{marginal utility of OG})_A = (\text{marginal utility of OG})_B$

Employing (7) to simplify (6),

$$(8)\ \frac{BB'}{AA'} = \frac{(\text{marginal utility of income})_A}{(\text{marginal utility of income})_B}$$

Equation (8) restates the Aaron and McGuire theorem, that is, that benefits should be imputed to each household in proportion to the reciprocal of its marginal utility of income.

Several additional assumptions are required in order to be able to employ the Aaron and McGuire method to allocate the benefits across income classes.[45] First, the relationship between the total money value of use-of-income benefits and government expenditures must be determined. As mentioned earlier, total government expenditures will equal the total money value of use-of-income benefits only if it can be assumed that provision of the service is optimal (Σ MRS=MC) and that the cost of providing the service is constant. If this is true then:

$$(1)\ (MRS^A)\ (OG) + (MRS^B)\ (OG) = E$$

where E represents total expenditure for the public good and MRS^A and MRS^B represent the marginal rates of substitution for A and B, respectively, or the slopes of $A'C_A$ and $B'C_B$ in Figure 3.

Restating (7) above in terms of the partial derivatives of U^A and U^B with respect to OG,

$$(2) \qquad \frac{\partial u^A}{\partial OG} = \frac{\partial u^B}{\partial OG} = C.$$

Since $MRS^A = \dfrac{\dfrac{\partial u^A}{\partial OG}}{MU_Y^A}$ and $MRS^B = \dfrac{\dfrac{\partial u^B}{\partial OG}}{MU_Y^B}$

where MU_Y^A and MU_Y^B represent the partial derivatives of U^A and U^B with respect to gross personal income (Y), then

$$(3) \qquad \frac{MRS^A}{MRS^B} = \frac{\dfrac{\partial u^A/\partial OG}{MU_Y^A}}{\dfrac{\partial u^B/\partial OG}{MU_Y^B}}$$

$$(4) \quad MRS^A. \ MU_Y^A = MRS^B. \ MU_Y^B = C.$$

$$(5) \qquad \text{a.} \quad MRS^A = \frac{C}{MU_Y^A}$$

$$\qquad \text{b.} \quad MRS^B = \frac{C}{MU_Y^B}$$

By substituting (5) into (1) the value of the public good consumed by each individual may be stated as follows:

$$(6) \quad \frac{C}{MU_Y^A} \cdot OG + \frac{C}{MU_Y^B} \cdot OG = E$$

Fraction of the total value of public good consumed by A	+	Fraction of the total value of public good consumed by B	=	E

Therefore, since E is known, it can be imputed to individuals by income class, if the functional relationship between marginal utility and income can be specified.

The functional relationship between marginal utility and income

Aaron and McGuire show that the selection of a utility function critically influences the allocation of benefits of public goods across income classes. Both they[46] and Greene, Neenan, and Scott[47] provide numerical examples illustrating the sensitivity of the results to the form of utility function chosen. For example, assuming three different utility functions with implied marginal utilities of: $MU_y = K$, $MU_y = \frac{K}{Y}$, $MU_y = \frac{K}{Y^2}$, Greene, Neenan, and Scott employ the procedures developed above to show how the distribution of \$500 of use-of-income benefits would vary between two individuals with incomes of \$1,000 and \$2,000 respectively. They assume that the two individuals have identical, separable utility functions and that total government outlays equal total use-of-income benefits. The results are illustrated in Table 1; these indicate that according to functions two and three, with the marginal utility of income declining proportionately with income and in proportion to the square of income, respectively, the higher income individual is imputed larger benefits than the lower income individual. These results illustrate Pigou's point that whether imputed benefits from a public good, expressed as a fraction of income, rise or fall with income, depends upon the *rate* at which marginal utility diminishes.[48]

Measuring the relationship between marginal utility and income has been attempted by a number of well known economists over a period of many years. Irving Fisher, in a study concerned with the problems of tax incidence and equity, appears to have been the first.[49] Ragnar Frisch was also a pioneer in the measurement of the income elasticity of marginal utility which he considered as the flexibility of marginal utility.[50] Frisch thought that in estimating this crucial parameter, cardinal utility had been brought back to life. However, Sato later showed that the parameter estimated by Frisch only describes the curvature of indifference curves and therefore does not have any intrinsic cardinal properties.[51]

Maital has examined recent empirical estimates of the income elasticity of marginal utility and supports a particular estimate of this parameter for the United States. In his analysis, he employs the following general marginal utility function:

$$MU(Y) = KY^{-\emptyset}$$

where ϕ represents the elasticity of marginal utility with respect to income.[52] ϕ also may be interpreted as the inverse of the elasticity of substitution between goods.[53] For this reason, Maital was able to extract values for ϕ from international estimates of the elasticity of substitution among goods.[54] The sample included eight countries and yielded the following estimates of ϕ: 1.04 for the United Kingdom, 1.46 for Japan, 1.50 for the United States, 1.55 for Canada, 1.85-2.13 for Norway, 2.35 for Australia, 2.16, 3.14, and 2.84 for the Netherlands, based upon separate studies, and 2.85 for Israel. The value of 1.50 for the United States was based upon a study by Powell, Van Hoa, and Wilson.[55] Two other independent studies by Mera[56] and Fellner,[57] using different methodologies, also estimated a value of 1.50 for the United States. Mera attempted to determine the form of the marginal utility function implied by effective income tax payments in relation to income in the United States during the period 1948 to 1968, if it were assumed that the U.S. personal income tax structure were designed to exact equal absolute amounts of utility from each taxpayer.

TABLE 1: Distribution of use-of-income benefits under three different utility assumptions

	Use-of-Income Benefits	
Utility Assumptions	**Individual A Income = \$1,000**	**Individual B Income = \$2,000**
1. $MU_y = K$	250.00	250.00
2. $MU_y = \frac{K}{Y}$	166.67	333.33
3. $MU_y = \frac{K}{Y^2}$	100.00	400.00

Source: Greene, Neenan, and Scott, *Fiscal Interactions in a Metropolitan Area*, p. 44.

Fellner's method of estimating the elasticity of marginal utility with respect to income is similar to that of Irving Fisher and represents a clear exposition of the problem. It may be summarized as follows: Assume that a given utility-maximizing individual with a given income purchases X_1 of commodity 1 at price p_1. P_1 is raised by K percent and the individual is compensated with sufficient additional income to induce him to continue purchasing X_1. The percentage increase in income is recorded. Fellner, assuming separability, that is, that the utility derived from one good is unaffected by other goods consumed, shows how the elasticity of marginal utility with respect to income may be determined by first stating the first order condition for utility maximization:

$$\frac{\partial u/\partial x_1}{p_1} = \lambda, \text{ where}$$

λ = the marginal utility of income, or MU_y
x_1 = the commodity
p_1 = the price of the commidity
and $\frac{\partial u}{\partial x_1}$ = the marginal utility of X_1

Since the marginal utility of x_1 or $\frac{\partial u}{\partial x_1}$ remains the same at both the lower and the higher price, and the price of x_1 has increased by K percent, then the first order condition ". . . tells us that the marginal utility of income (or of the dollar) in the high-income situation is k% lower than in the low-income situation."[58] Therefore, since the percentage change of both income and marginal utility are both known, the elasticity of marginal utility with respect to income may be computed.

Several questions may be raised regarding Maital's proposed 1.50 estimate of $\emptyset$ for the United States based upon the identical estimates provided in the three studies mentioned above.[59] First, in both the Fellner study and that by Powell, Van Hoa, and Wilson, separable utility functions were assumed; second, private rather than public sector data were employed in both of those studies; finally, the Mera study is based upon the improbable assumption, mentioned above, that the federal income tax structure in the United States was designed to exact equal absolute amounts of utility from each taxpayer. When separable utility functions are assumed, the inverse of the elasticity of substitution between goods may be interpreted as the elasticity of marginal utility with respect to income. However, a change in the inverse of the elasticity of substitution among goods can be considered an accurate measure of the change in the marginal utility of real income only if two goods are neither substitutes nor complements. If publicly and privately provided services were complements, then as the consumption of publicly provided services increases, the marginal utility of privately provided services tends to increase, and the change in the inverse of the marginal rate of substitution among goods would over-estimate any decrease in the marginal utility of income; if the two services were substitutes, any decrease in the marginal utility of income would be underestimated.

Maital argues that the assumption of separable utility for privately and publicly provided services is necessary in order to facilitate empirical work and that unrealistic assumptions are almost always necessary in order to apply theory to reality. He finds separability an acceptable compromise solution to the question of whether public and private goods are complements or substitutes until further research becomes available.[60]

The Willingness-to-Pay approach for imputing use-of-income benefits to income classes

In 1844, Jules Dupuit argued that the evaluation of government services needs to be placed on a "willingness-to-pay" basis:

> To sum up, political economy has to take as the measure of the utility of an object the maximum sacrifice which each consumer would be willing to make in order to acquire the object . . . . Thus when a bridge is built and the state establishes a tariff, the latter is not related to cost of production: the heavy cart is charged less than the sprung carriage even though it causes more wear to the timber of the carriage-way. Why are there two different prices for the same service? Because the poor man does not attach the same value to crossing the bridge as the rich man does, and raising the charge would only prevent him from crossing. Canal and railway tariffs differentiate between the various classes of goods and passengers, and lay down markedly different rates for them although the costs are more or less the same . . . . The purchaser never pays more for the product than the value he places on its utility.[61]

Greene, Neenan, and Scott employ a willingness-to-pay approach in imputing use-of-income benefits to income classes. They adopt the general functional form for allocating benefits from pure public goods employed by Maital, that is $MU(Y) = KY^{-\phi}$;[62] however, they assume an elasticity of marginal utility with respect to income of 1.0, which they derive from the willingness to pay for public services as expressed in survey and voting data, rather than a value of 1.5, which is supported by Maital.[63] They argue that subfederal public services, which are the subject of their study, generally tend to *complement*, rather than substitute for, privately provided services. Therefore, the value of $\emptyset$ used to evaluate publicly provided services would be expected to be less than 1.50.

Applying Fellner's analysis to the public sector and using survey and voting data, they derive an estimate of $\emptyset$ for evaluating public output.[64] First, if the given individual's tax price were doubled and the marginal utility of x_1 remained constant, the marginal utility of income would be one-half of its former value. Second, in order to maintain the marginal utility of x_1 constant, that is, induce the individual to willingly finance or demand the same level of public service as he had before his tax price was doubled, evidence from survey and voting data, discussed further below, indicates that his income would have to be doubled. Finally, since the marginal utility of income is reduced by one-half when income is doubled in the above example, the elasticity of marginal utility with respect to income, or $\emptyset$ in Maital's general expression for the marginal utility of income ($MU(Y) = KY^{-\emptyset}$) is equal to one. A value of 1.0 for $\emptyset$ also will be used in the empirical section of this study.

Neenan supported the hypothesis that citizens' willingness to pay for publicly provided services would be proportional to income, if tax incidence were proportional, with evidence from various voting and attitude surveys, four of which are discussed below.[65] Of these, three concern local government services in the United States, financed by property taxes, and the fourth concerns publicly provided services in Basel-Stadt, one of the Swiss cantons, financed by a progressive tax structure. The three studies concerned with public services in the United States by Boskoff and Ziegler,[66] Watson[67] and Wilson and Banfield[68] each provided similar results. In both the Boskoff and Ziegler and Watson studies, there was a positive correlation between income and support for each of the expenditure items included in the survey and support tended to increase sharply with each succeeding income class. Therefore, given the tax structure in each of these localities, higher income individuals indicated a greater willingness to pay for increased public services than low and middle income individuals. Banfield and Wilson also found a consistently more favorable attitude over rising income classes; in contrast to the Watson and Boskoff and Ziegler studies, however, they found that support rose as described only after the lowest income class. Their results indicated that the percent-yes vote in the lowest income wards and precincts ranged from 75 to 90 percent, but declined sharply over middle income groups; in the highest income districts, support for the measures increased again to the range found among the lowest income groups, although these "would give them only trivial benefits while imposing substantial costs upon them."[69]

Willingness to pay for a public service is clearly a function of both an individual's attitude toward the public service and his anticipated tax liability, that is, his "fiscal residuum." Neenan defines the concept of a fiscal residuum as "the difference, expressed in welfare terms, between a person's perceived benefits and perceived tax liability of any budgetary adjustment."[70] He interprets the pattern of support that was summarized above as follows:

> 1. Very low income voters perceive positive benefits with a negligible anticipated tax liability from proposed budgetary actions. Thus their perceived fiscal residua is positive and they favor the proposals.
> 2. Middle income voters may indeed perceive benefits from proposed budgetary action, but above a certain income threshhold their anticipated disutility from increased taxes is likewise significant. Often, therefore, this group faces negative fiscal residua from proposed actions and hence opposes them.
> 3. Higher income voters have a more favorable attitude toward increased expenditures because they evaluate benefits, especially redistributive benefits, more favorably than do middle income families. This disposition coupled with the regressive incidence of most local tax structures tend to generate positive fiscal residua for high income groups.[71]

As mentioned above, Neenan attributes the strong support for public programs among higher income groups to the regressive impact of local tax structures, particularly the property tax, which was to finance these programs.[72] He suggests that "if, for example, a proportional or progressive tax structure were substituted for the currently regressive structure, we would expect the percent-yes vote in referenda generally to shift upward across lower income classes and fall in the higher income classes."[73]

Results of the Frey and Kohn analysis of public finance referenda in Basel-Stadt, Switzerland, appear to confirm Neenan's expectation.[74] Whereas the results in the three studies for the United States were approximately a U-shaped function of family income, the percent-yes vote was found to be more or less constant across all income classes in Basel-Stadt, with the exception of the lowest income class, where the percent-yes vote was higher. Neenan attributes the difference between the results for the United States in the studies reviewed and those for Basel-Stadt to the difference in the tax structures of the localities involved.[75]

In summary, in the willingness-to-pay approach, the method developed by Aaron and McGuire is applied to impute use-of-income benefits by income class using the general functional form for the marginal utility of income proposed by Maital and a value for $\emptyset$ that is estimated on the basis of Fellner's analysis and survey and voting data as equal to 1.0. Greene, Neenan, and Scott employ this method not only to impute public non-redistributive and public redistributive use-of-income benefits but also to impute private use-of-income benefits by income class, after determining which income classes are the beneficiaries of the public service in question. (See Figure 1.) They argue that "in actuality all major public services generate benefits in a more or less ill-defined manner for the population at large even though some services, say public education, also provide benefits for an identifiable group. Thus all public services properly fall within the domain of Samuelson's recent definition of a "public good as 'one that enters two or more person's utility'."[76] Neenan also has defended the treatment of all publicly provided services as pure public goods by arguing that:

> In a competitive market a consumer maximizes utility by adjusting the quantity of a commodity consumed, with the consequences that the marginal evaluation of any commodity tends to equal its market price and to be the same for all consumers. *In the public sector*, on the other hand, *a citizen is not free to adjust the quantity of public service consumed. As a result of this constraint, citizens marginal evaluations of a particular public service will only by chance tend to be the same.* Since citizen evaluations cannot be directly inferred from market values, some procedure for imputing benefits from public programs must be devised that is sensitive to the potential variation in citizens' marginal evaluations.[77] (Emphasis mine.)

The relationship between total government expenditures and total use-of-income benefits

In illustrating the Aaron and McGuire method for imputing the benefits from public services to individuals, it was assumed that the value of the public service to individuals equalled the cost of providing the service. It is not known, *a priori*, whether benefits exceed, fall short of, or equal the expenditures incurred to provide that service. This is a major theoretical problem!

Total government expenditures equal total marginal benefits produced by these expenditures only if (1) the public service is provided at an optimal level, and (2) the marginal cost of providing the service is constant. Both of these conditions are represented in Figure 4 below.[78]

Optimal provision of a public service

Pareto optimal output is achieved at the level at which the sum of the marginal rates of substitution across all individuals equals the marginal cost of the public good. In Figure 4, a community of three individuals, A, B, and C, is represented, each of whom is to remain on indifference curves U_A, U_B, and U_C, respectively. The production transformation curve between public and private output is represented by TT′ and is constructed to indicate constant marginal costs of provision. The socially optimal level of the public good is provided at Q; if output exceeds Q, then marginal cost exceeds the summed marginal rates of substitution and total costs exceed total benefits; if output falls short of Q, then marginal cost is less than the summed marginal rates of substitution and total costs are less than total benefits. The value of the public service, evaluated at the margin, only equals the product of the marginal rate of substitution or the slope of TT′ (which equals the marginal cost of the Qth unit or the [tax] price) and Q units at output Q.

Greene has examined several models of the city decision-making process and the implications of these for the relationship between the marginal benefits and the marginal cost of a collective service.[79] For example, Figure 5 illustrates the model discussed by Aaron and McGuire,[80] and Greene suggests that it might represent the imposition of an optimal social welfare criterion by an omniscient and benevolent dictator. T_R, T_S, and T_O represent the tax prices per unit of service provided for residents, suburbanites and others outside of the urban area, respectively, and the marginal cost of providing a unit of the service equals the sum of T_R, T_S, and T_O. The demand curve, or marginal evaluation, for the given public service is represented by ME_R, ME_S and ME_O for each of these groups, respectively. At Q_O, where Σ ME = MC, output is optimally provided; although the sum of the marginal evaluation equals the marginal cost of providing the service at the margin, however, the marginal evaluation of each of the respective groups may equal, exceed, or fall short of, its own tax price.

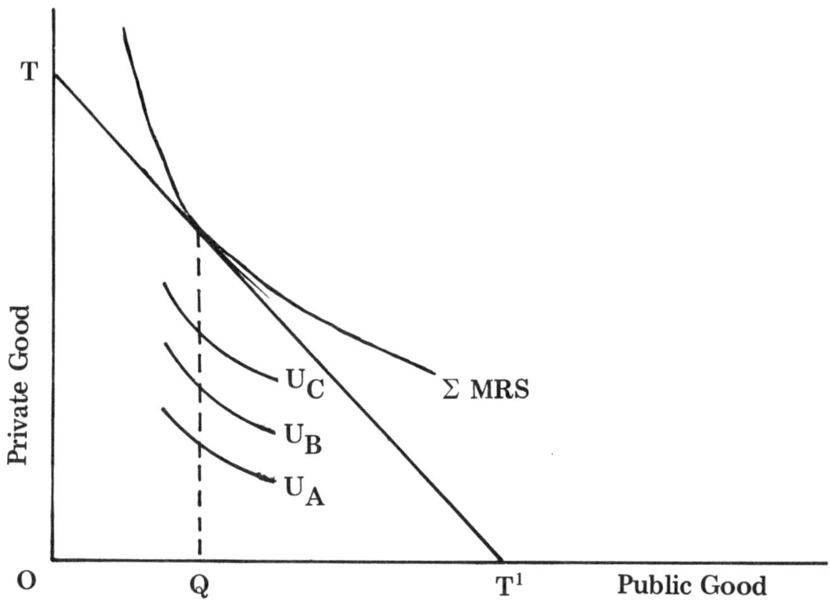

FIGURE 4: Illustration of the two conditions which must be fulfilled for total government expenditures to equal total marginal benefits received by individuals: (1) optimal provision of public services and (2) constant marginal cost of provision.

Source: Greene, Neenan, and Scott, *Fiscal Interactions in a Metropolitan Area*, p. 52

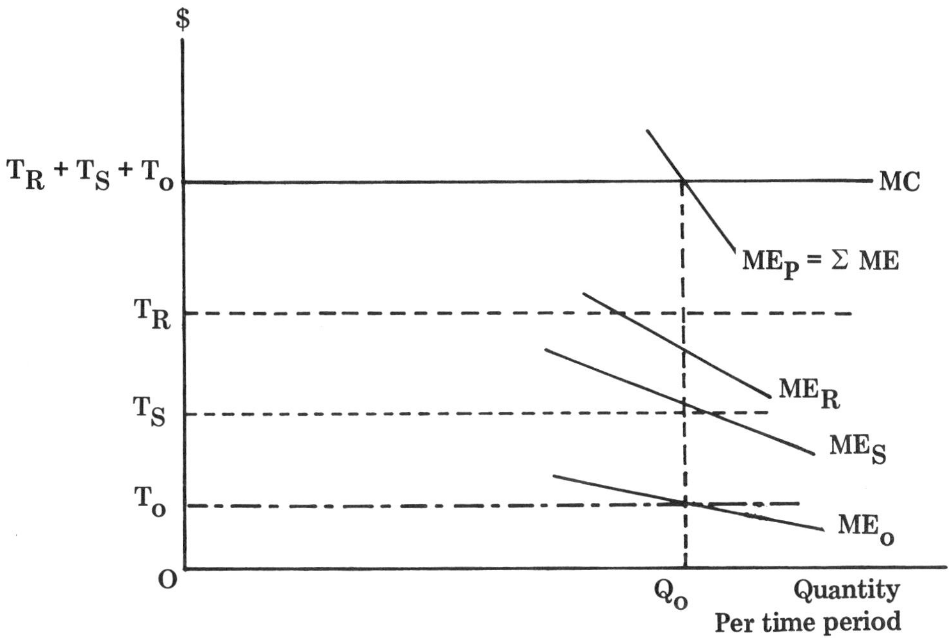

FIGURE 5: Model of an optimal social welfare criterion imposed by an omniscient and benevolent dictator.

Source: Greene, "Collective Decision-Making Models and the Measurement of Benefits in Fiscal Incidence Studies," p. 180.

Greene also considers a model involving a purely democratic decision-making process in which individuals differ and the median or representative voter controls the output level chosen. The community consists of three individuals, A, B, and C, preferring an output level of Q_A, Q_B, and Q_C, respectively, as shown in Figure 6. Greene concludes that without empirical evidence, there is no *a priori* reason to believe that the output level chosen, Q_B, will exceed or fall short of the city's optimum output level of Q_R, unless transaction and bargaining costs between groups within the city are zero. Since there is no reason to believe that the city's optimum output level exceeds or falls short of the social optimum, there is no reason to assume that the social optimum output level exceeds or falls short of the output level selected; therefore, there is no reason to believe that summed marginal evaluations exceed or fall short of MC.[81]

Greene, Neenan, and Scott also employ a democratic, individualistic majority-voting-rule model in their study and derive hypotheses regarding the optimality of public output.[82] However, the analysis did not permit them to conclude that public services generally were provided at an optimal, suboptimal, or superoptimal level. They suggest that if this were to be attempted for a specific case study of public services provided by local governments, it would be necessary to know the income elasticities of the tax structure; the income elasticities of demand for the public service; the economic rent received by residents of an urban area from local government expenditures; and the tax payments of non-residents to the local government as well as the benefits received from the services provided by the local government. In particular, the magnitude and the distribution of decision-making costs would need to be examined in order to determine the effect of these on the level of output. Without strong evidence indicating that output was either suboptimal or superoptimal, Greene, Neenan, and Scott assumed in their analysis that output tended to be close to the social optimum.

Non-constant costs

If output is supplied at the socially optimal level, the total budgetary cost of providing the service will only equal total benefits to individuals if marginal cost and average cost are equal. The total budgetary cost of providing the given service will exceed total benefits to individuals if average costs are falling; they will fall short of total benefits to individuals if average costs are rising. This is a particularly difficult problem, since many public services are thought to involve decreasing costs. It has been suggested that in cases of

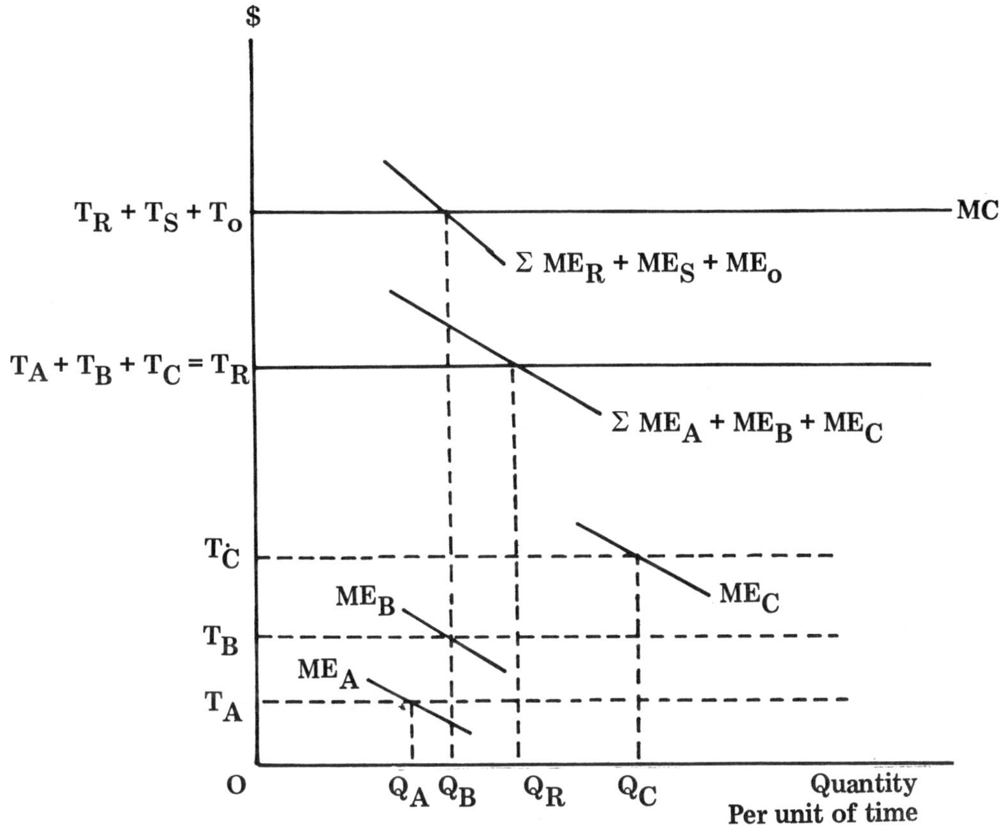

FIGURE 6: Individualistic collective decision-making model: a purely democratic decision-making process is assumed in which individuals differ and the output level is controlled by the median or representative voter.

Source: Greene, "Collective Decision-Making Models and the Measurement of Benefits in Fiscal Incidence Studies," p. 183.

decreasing costs, the consumer surplus involved might be estimated, as in cost-benefit analysis; however, this would not be consistent with the objective of placing the valuation of publicly provided services on the same basis as privately provided services.[83] Furthermore, in cases of increasing costs, this approach might result in an overestimation of benefits.

Use-of-Income benefits provided by investment expenditures

Different approaches need to be developed for benefit incidence analysis of current and investment expenditures. Benefit incidence studies attempt to allocate the benefits from government expenditures to income classes in a given period of time. While consumption expenditures generate benefits in the period in which they are incurred, investment expenditures generate benefits in future years.

Theoretical contributions to cost benefit analysis may provide some guidelines as to the directions that future research should take concerning the incidence of public investment expenditures. Feldstein, for example, developed a theoretical technique for analyzing the benefits from a particular project by calculating its Net Social Benefit (NSB), which he defined as the net addition to consumption expected as a result of undertaking the project.[84] Two models were presented for calculating the social opportunity cost (SOC) of funds employed. His exposition may be summarized as follows: When the government transfers resources from the private to the public sector during the life of a project, consumption is foregone. The current value of all consumption that is foregone is calculated using a social-time-preference (STP) discount rate in order to make intertemporal comparisons of social benefits and costs. The STP discount rate is a normative interest rate, reflecting society's evaluation of the relative desirability of consumption at different points in time. The SOC of funds transferred from the private to the public sector is then the current value of the aggregate consumption time-stream that is foregone as a result of the transfer. When funds are transferred from the private to the public sector, it may be assumed that private consumption and private investment are decreased. The original private investment would have generated an income stream for investors and workers, part of which would have been consumed and the rest reinvested. The reinvested funds would have generated a further income stream, part of which would again have been consumed and the rest reinvested. Feldstein defines the current or discounted value (using the STP rate to discount) of the aggregate consumption time-stream that the original investment would have provided as the private investment multiplier M. He develops a simplified model to demonstrate how M might be estimated:

$$(1)\ M = \sum_{t=1}^{\infty} \frac{Ct}{(1 + d)^{t}} ,$$

where C_t represents consumption in year t resulting from income of Y_t received in year t and d represents the social time preference rate (STP). (In the following equations, Feldstein attempts to express C_t in terms of variables that are known.)

$$(2)\ C_t = mY_t \quad (t = 1, \ldots),$$

where m represents the marginal propensity to consume.

$$(3)\ Y_t = \frac{r}{x} \sum_{n=o}^{t-1} I_n \quad (t = 1, \ldots),$$

where Y_t represents income received from investment in year zero; I_n represents investment in year t out of Y_t received; r represents the marginal rate of return to private investors; x represents the proportion of the increased national income generated by marginal investments that is received by private investors. Therefore, in Feldstein's example, a 1£ investment generates a total direct increase in income which equals an annual income stream of £ (r/x).

$$(4)\ I_t = Y_t - C_t = (1\text{-}m)\ Y_t \quad (t = 1, \ldots).$$

From equations (2), (3) and (4),

$$(5)\ C_t = \frac{mr}{x} \left[1 + r/_x\ (1\text{-}m) \right]^{t-1} \quad (t = 1, \ldots).$$

Substituting (5) into (1),

$$(6)\ M = \frac{mr}{x} \sum_{t\text{-}1}^{\infty} \frac{\left[1 + (r/_x)\ (1\text{-}m)\right]^{t-1}}{(1 + d)^{t}}$$

Feldstein also develops a second, more realistic model, wherein he disaggregates the consumption function and incorporates a tax function.

Using the parameter M, the NSB, or the value of the net addition to future consumption that the project would produce then may be determined. The NSB is calculated as the difference between the discounted value of the time stream of consumption provided (B_c) and the discounted value of the time stream of consumption foregone (SOC): NSB = B_c - SOC.

Summary

In this chapter, contributions to the development of the theory of benefit incidence were discussed. First, an outline of the benefits generated for individuals by government expenditures was presented in Figure 1. As shown in the diagram, government expenditures may affect an individual's welfare through the effects of the expenditures themselves on his sources of income and by providing him with consumer satisfaction through the use of his income to purchase public services. These two types of benefits were classified as source-of-income benefits and use-of-income benefits, respectively. How benefits are *defined* and *measured* are important and difficult questions in any analysis of benefit incidence! The discussion then focused upon theoretically appropriate methods for evaluating the various benefits classfied as either source-of-income or use-of-income benefits in Figure 1. The theoretical discussion was complemented with comments upon both the feasibility of measuring these benefits as the theory suggests and attempts that have been made to empirically measure the benefits involved. The main conclusions of this analysis are summarized below.

Source-of-income benefits may be in the form of money transfers, in-kind transfers, and net increases in income due to general equilibrium adjustments initiated by government purchases of factors of production. Theoretically, the net benefit from money transfers should equal the sum of the value of the money transfer and the value of increased leisure time less the income that would have been earned if the transfer had not been made. However, the full cash value of money transfers generally is taken as a measure of the net benefit, due to the practical difficulties involved in estimating these adjustments. Similarly, the welfare gain to recipients of in-kind transfers (or transfers received by lower income citizens who have not incurred any tax liability *qua* recipients of the transfers) may not be equal to their cost because, for example, they constrain consumption choices which would be available if cash transfers were provided. However, due to the lack of empirical research on how to adjust the value of in-kind transfers to money equivalents, the cost of providing these also is taken as a measure of benefits. Finally, the net income gains or losses due to factor payments by government should be measured by comparing salary payments made to government employees with what the same employees would have obtained if government had not incurred the expenditure. The magnitude of the net gain to a public employee would depend upon whether there were full or less than full employment in the economy. Estimation of these effects generally is not attempted in benefit incidence studies.

Use-of-income benefits, also known as taxpayer benefits, include both direct and indirect benefits to recipients.[85] Depending upon the nature of the public service, it may generate any, all, or any combination of the following three types of benefits: (1) private benefits for direct recipients, (2) public non-redistributive benefits for society as a whole, without regard to income, and (3) public redistributive benefits to the non-poor or non-recipient taxpayers who are willing and able to finance redistributive programs. If redistributive programs are optimally provided, total public redistributive benefits should equal the total absolute value of money and in-kind transfers.

Imputation of use-of-income benefits to income classes needs to be based upon a method that reflects citizens' marginal evaluations of the benefits generated by public services. Aaron and McGuire developed a theoretically defensible procedure for evaluating and imputing the benefits from pure public goods to income classes. Assuming that all households have identical and separable utility functions for public and private goods, that each household is provided the same amount of a given public good, and that total government expenditures for the public good equal total benefits generated, they show that: (1) the "value in exchange" of the public good to each household equals the product of its marginal rate of substitution and the amount of public good provided; and that (2) each household may be imputed a share of the total benefits generated by the public good in inverse proportion to its marginal utility of income. They also showed that the allocation of benefits to income classes is highly sensitive to the values that are either explicitly or implicitly assigned to the marginal utility of income. In order to employ this procedure to impute benefits across income classes, therefore, particular values for the marginal utility of income need to be specified.

In the "willingness-to-pay" procedure for analyzing benefit incidence, the Aaron and McGuire method is employed to impute all use-of-income benefits to income classes. The general functional form proposed by Maital, namely, $MU(Y) = KY^{-\emptyset}$, is adopted, and a value for $\emptyset$, the income elasticity of marginal utility with respect to income, is estimated on the basis of Fellner's analysis complemented with survey and voting data. Fellner's analysis, using the first order condition for utility maximization, showed that if the tax price for a public service were doubled and the individual's income were increased sufficiently to induce him to finance the same level of public output, the marginal utility of income at the higher income level would have one-half the value it had at the lower income level; voting and survey data indicate that his income would have to be doubled in order to induce him to finance the same output level, if his tax price were doubled. Therefore, a value of 1.0 for $\emptyset$ was assumed by Greene, Neenan, and Scott in imputing all use-of-income benefits according to the willingness-to-pay approach. Neenan, in an earlier study, referred to this parameter as the "willingness-to-pay, or effective demand index of the benefits from public services."[86]

The chapter also included a discussion of the implications of the assumption that total use-of-income benefits equal total government expenditures for a given public service. It was pointed out that for this to be true, the service must be optimally supplied and the marginal cost of providing the service must be constant. In previous benefit incidence studies, determining whether public services are underprovided or overextended generally has not been attempted.

Finally, the issue of how to impute use-of-income benefits from investment expenditures was discussed briefly. Asset creating or investment expenditures generate use-of-income benefits not only in the year in which the expenditure is incurred, but also in later years. Theoretical contributions to cost-benefit analysis may provide some guidelines for future research into this unresolved issue in benefit incidence theory. Feldstein's theoretical technique for determining the net addition to consumption as a result of public investments was summarized and presented as an illustration.

NOTES AND REFERENCES

[1] International Bank for Reconstruction and Development, *World Bank Atlas: Population, Per Capita Product and Growth Rates* (Washington, D.C.: International Bank for Reconstruction and Development, 1974).

[2] Richard A. Musgrave and Malcolm Gillis (eds.), *Fiscal Reform for Colombia, Final Report and Staff Papers of the Colombian Commission on Tax Reform* (Cambridge, Massachusetts: Harvard Law School International Tax Program, 1971).

[3] Vito Tanzi, "Fiscal Reform for Colombia: The Report of the Musgrave Commission," *Inter-American Economic Affairs* 26 (Summer 1972): 80.

[4] R. M. Bird and L. De Wulf, "Taxation and Income Distribution in Latin America: A Critical Review of Empirical Studies," IMF *Staff Papers* 20 (November 1973): 672-73.

[5] Robert S. McNamara, president, World Bank Group, "Address to the Board of Governors," IBRD/IMF Annual Meeting, Washington, D.C., 25 September 1972 (Washington, D.C.: International Bank for Reconstruction and Development, 1972), p. 17.

[6] Charles E. McLure, Jr., "On the Theory and Methodology of Estimating Benefit and Expenditure Incidence," paper presented at the Workshop on "Income Distribution and Its Role in Development," William Marsh Rice University, Houston, Texas, 26 April 1974, pp. 5-6. (Xeroxed.)

[7] *Ibid.*, p. 2.

[8] See, for example, James M. Buchanan, *Public Finance in Democratic Process: Fiscal Institutions and Individual Choice* (Chapel Hill: The University of North Carolina Press, 1967), pp. 11-12.

[9] The individualistic or self-interest approach is opposed in the literature by those supporting the "public interest" approach, also labelled the "organic" approach. The public interest approach is based upon the assumption that the collectivity has concerns that extend beyond the aggregate preferences or values of individual citizens; however, the nature of the objective function is not clearly specified. The individualistic approach is more elegant and rigorous. Furthermore, it can be both narrowly formulated in terms of consumer preference or broadened to include social and political values. For a critical discussion of both approaches, see: Jesse Burkhead and Jerry Miner, *Public Expenditure* (Chicago: Aldine-Atherton, 1971), pp. 145-71.

[10] The recent study by: Kenneth V. Greene, William B. Neenan, and Claudia D. Scott, *Fiscal Interactions in a Metropolitan Area* (Lexington, Massachusetts: Lexington Books, 1974), goes beyond all previous benefit incidence studies. With some modifications, the framework and procedures which they have proposed have been adopted in this study.

[11] *Ibid.*, p. 32.

[12] M. Schmundt, E. Smolensky, and L. Stiefel, *The Evaluation by Recipients of In-Kind Transfers* (Madison: University of Wisconsin, Institute for Research on Poverty, 1974), p. 3.

[13] Charles E. McLure, Jr., "The Theory of Expenditure Incidence," *Finanzarchiv* 30 (1972): 432-53.

[14] Greene, Neenan, and Scott, *op. cit.*, p. 30.

[15] Richard A. Musgrave, "Provision of Social Goods," in *Public Economics*, edited by J. Margolis and H. Guitton (London: Macmillan, 1969), p. 125.

[16] Samuelson has suggested that most of the public services which are neither purely private nor purely public be formally regarded as belonging in the public-good category. Therefore, he has proposed the following definition of a public good: "A public good is one that enters two or more persons' utility." See Paul A. Samuelson, "Pure Theory of Public Expenditure and Taxation," in *Public Economics*, p. 108.

[17] McLure refers to these as taxpayer benefits in: McLure, "On the Theory and Methodology of Estimating Benefit and Expenditure Incidence," p. 34; Greene, Neenan, and Scott classify them as public redistributive benefits in: Greene, Neenan, and Scott, *op. cit.*, p. 42.

[18] Kenneth E. Boulding, "Notes on a Theory of Philanthropy," in *Philanthropy and Public Policy*, edited by Frank G. Dickinson (New York: National Bureau of Economic Research, 1962), p. 61.

[19] *Ibid.*, pp. 59-61.

[20] Thomas R. Ireland, *The Economics of Charity* (Blacksburg: Center for the Study of Public Choice, 1970), p. 22.

[21] Frances Fox Piven and Richard A. Cloward, *Regulating the Poor* (New York: Pantheon Books, 1971), p. XIII.

[22] William S. Vickrey, "One Economist's View of Philanthropy," in *Philanthropy and Public Policy*, ed. Frank G. Dickinson (New York: National Bureau of Economic Research, 1962), p. 41; and Stephen A. Marglin, "The Social Rate of Discount and the Optimal Rate of Investment," *Quarterly Journal of Economics* 77 (1963): 95-111.

[23] Vickrey, "One Economist's View of Philanthropy," pp. 41-42.

[24] Harold M. Hochman and James D. Rodgers, "Utility Interdependence and Income Transfers Through Charity," in *Transfers in an Urbanized Economy*, ed. Kenneth E. Boulding, Martin Pfaff, and Anita Pfaff (Belmont: Wadsworth, 1973), pp. 63-77.

[25] William Watts and Lloyd A. Free, *State of the Nation* (New York: Universe Books, 1973), pp. 320-33.

[26] Harold M. Hochman and James D. Rodgers, "Pareto Optimal Redistribution," *American Economic Review* 61 (1969): 543.

[27] *Ibid.*, p. 542.

[28] See *Ibid.*, p. 545.

[29] *Ibid.*, p. 553.

[30] *Ibid.*, p. 555.

[31] See R.S. Goldfarb, "Pareto Optimal Redistribution: Comment," *The American Economic Review* 60 (December 1970): 994-96; Greene, Neenan, and Scott, *op. cit.*, 39; P. A. Meyer and J. J. Shipley, "Pareto Optimal Redistribution: Comment," *The American Econom-*

ic Review 60 (December 1970); 988-90; E. J. Mishan, "The Futility of Pareto-Efficient Distributions," *The American Economic Review* 62 (December 1972): 971-976; R. A. Musgrave, "Pareto Optimal Redistribution: Comment," *The American Economic Review* 60 (December 1970): 991-93.

[32] Mishan, "The Futility of Pareto-Efficient Distributions," *op. cit.*, pp. 974-75.

[33] *Ibid.*, p. 976.

[34] Musgrave, "Pareto Optimal Redistribution: Comment," *op. cit.*, p. 991.

[35] Harold M. Hochman and James D. Rodgers, "Pareto Optimal Redistribution: Reply," *The American Economic Review*, 60 (December 1970): 998-999.

[36] Greene, Neenan, and Scott, *op. cit.*, p. 39.

[37] Henry Aaron and Martin McGuire, "Public Goods and Income Distribution," *Econometrica* 38 (November 1970): 907-14.

[38] Ugo Mazzola, "The Formation of the Prices of Public Goods," (1890) in *Classics in the Theory of Public Finance* ed. Richard A. Musgrave and Alan T. Peacock, trans. Elizabeth Henderson (London: Macmillan & Co. Ltd., 1962), pp. 37-47.

[39] Erik Lindahl, "Just Taxation—a Positive Solution," (1919) in *Ibid.*, trans. by Elizabeth Henderson, pp. 168-76; and *Idem*, "Some Controversial Questions in the Theory of Taxation," in *Ibid.*, trans. by Elizabeth Henderson, pp. 214-32.

[40] Aaron and McGuire, *op. cit.*, p. 911. The authors state that assumptions (3) to (8) could be eliminated if information supporting some other relation became available or if another assumption appeared preferable.

[41] Shlomo Maital, "Public Goods and Income Distribution: Some Further Results," *Econometrica* 41 (May 1973): 561-63.

[42] Aaron and McGuire, *op. cit.*, p. 909.

[43] Aaron and McGuire, *op. cit.*, p. 909.

[44] Maital, *op. cit.*, pp. 562-64.

[45] The following procedures illustrating the Aaron and McGuire method were drawn from: Greene, Neenan, and Scott, *op. cit.*, pp. 43-44.

[46] Aaron and McGuire, *op. cit.*, pp. 914-19.

[47] Greene, Neenan, and Scott, *op. cit.*, pp. 44-45.

[48] A. C. Pigou, *A Study in Public Finance*, rev. 3d ed. (London: Macmillan and Co. Ltd., 1962), p. 111.

[49] Irving Fisher, "A Statistical Method for Measuring 'Marginal Utility' and Testing the Justice of a Progressive Income Tax," in *Economic Essays, Contributed in Honor of John Bates Clark* edited

by Jacob H. Hollander (New York: The Macmillan Company, 1927), pp. 157-93.

[50] Ragnar Frisch, "A Complete Scheme for Computing All Direct and Cross Demand Elasticities in a Model with Many Sectors," *Econometrica* 27 (1959): 177-96.

[51] Kazuo Sato, "Additive Utility Functions with Double-Log Consumer Demand Functions," *Journal of Political Economy* 80 (January/February 1972): 102-08.

[52] Maital, "Public Goods and Income Distribution: Some Further Results," pp. 564-67; and *Idem*, "Is Redistributive Taxation a Myth?" Discussion Paper No. 122, Institute of Economic Research, Queens University, Kingston, Ontario, January 1973, p. 5.

[53] Sato, *op. cit.*, p. 108.

[54] Maital, *op. cit.*, p. 8.

[55] Alan A. Powell, Tran Van Hoa, and R. H. Wilson, "A Multi-Sectoral Analysis of Consumer Demand in the Post-War Period," *The Southern Economic Journal* 35 (October 1968): 109-20.

[56] K. Mera, "Experimental Determination of Relative Marginal Utilities," *Quarterly Journal of Economics* 83 (August 1969): 464-77.

[57] William Fellner, "Operational Utility: The Theoretical Background and a Measurement," in *Ten Economic Studies in the Tradition of Irving Fisher* (New York: John Wiley & Sons, Inc., 1967), pp. 39-74.

[58] Fellner, *op. cit.*, pp. 48-49.

[59] The following points are discussed in: Greene, Neenan, and Scott, *op. cit.*, p. 46.

[60] Maital, *op. cit.*, p. 12.

[61] Jules Dupuit, "On the Measurement of the Utility of Public Works," in *Readings in Welfare Economics* ed. Kenneth J. Arrow and Tibor Scitovsky, trans. R. H. Barback (Homewood, Ill.: Irwin, 1969), pp. 261-62, quoted in William B. Neenan, *Political Economy of Urban Areas* (Chicago: Markham Publishing Company, 1972), pp. 85-86.

[62] Greene, Neenan, and Scott, *op. cit.*, p. 45.

[63] *Ibid.*, pp. 46-48.

[64] *Ibid.*

[65] Neenan, *op. cit.*, pp. 81-118.

[66] Alvin Boskoff and Harmon Ziegler, *Voting Patterns in a Local Election* (Philadelphia: Lippincott, 1964). The authors conducted a survey of voter attitudes in De Kalb County, Georgia, immediately after a $22 million bond referendum was held in 1961. Voters had approved all nine items with comfortable margins.

[67] Richard A. Watson, *The Politics of Urban Change* (Kansas

City: Community Studies, Inc., 1963). In this study, two groups of individuals were surveyed in Kansas City, Missouri, in order to determine citizens' willingness to pay higher taxes for increased public services: (1) middle income residents of an urban renewal project and (2) low income residents of an unrenewed, contiguous neighborhood.

[68] Edward C. Banfield and James Q. Wilson, "Voting Behaviour on Municipal Public Expenditures: A Study in Rationality and Self-Interest," in *The Public Economy of Urban Communities* (Washington, D.C.: Resources for the Future, 1975), pp. 74-91. The authors studied 35 referenda involving expenditure proposals during the period 1957 to 1963 in seven cities.

[69] Neenan, *op. cit.*, p. 99, quoting Banfield and Wilson, "Voting Behaviour on Municipal Public Expenditures: A Study in Rationality and Self-Interest," p. 79.

[70] *Ibid.*, p. 90.

[71] *Ibid.*, pp. 99-100.

[72] *Ibid.*, p. 102.

[73] *Ibid.*

[74] René L. Frey and Leopold Kohn, "An Economic Interpretation of Voting Behaviour on Public Finance Issues," *Kyklos* 23 (1970): 792-805. Frey and Kohn analyzed the results of 18 public finance referenda conducted in Basel-Stadt, Switzerland, during the period 1960 to 1969. Basel-Stadt has a population of 238,000 and is divided into 25 voting districts, each of which was classified according to its average personal income. Correlation coefficients were calculated between the average income per capita and the percent-yes vote in each district.

[75] Neenan, *op. cit.*, p. 102.

[76] Greene, Neenan, and Scott, *op. cit.*, p. 34; see also Paul A. Samuelson, "Pure Theory of Public Expenditure and Taxation," in *Public Economics*, p. 108.

[77] William B. Neenan, "Income Redistribution through Local Government Fiscs," Discussion Paper No. 290-75, Institute for Research on Poverty, University of Wisconsin, Madison, Wisconsin, July 1975, pp. 12-13.

[78] See Greene, Neenan, and Scott, *op. cit.*, pp. 51-52.

[79] Kenneth V. Greene, "Collective Decision-Making Models and the Measurement of Benefits in Fiscal Incidence Studies," *National Tax Journal* 26 (June 1973): 177-85.

[80] Aaron and McGuire, *op. cit.*

[81] Greene, "Collective Decision-Making Models," *op. cit.*, p. 183.

[82] Greene, Neenan, and Scott, *op. cit.*, pp. 51-60.

[83] For a brief discussion of this problem see: McLure, *op. cit.*, p. 53.

[84] Martin S. Feldstein, "Net Social Benefit Calculation and the Public Investment Decision," *Oxford Economic Papers* 16 (March 1964): 114-31.

[85] Government expenditures on education, for example, benefit families with children attending public schools; however, taxpayers without school children also may perceive benefits. They might support public schools either because they may in the future have children in school, because they have had children in school, because they believe that society as a whole benefits from having a literate population, or perhaps because they believe that the poor should have an opportunity to improve their status in society through education.

[86] Neenan, *Political Economy*, *op. cit.*, p. 83.

Chapter 2

BENEFITS FROM PUBLIC HEALTH EXPENDITURES

Introduction

Many of the most distinguished scholars in the field of economics have contributed to the development of concepts employed to measure the value of human capital produced by health services. Changes in the quality of people due to investments in education and health improve people as productive agents and yield a continuing stream of benefits in the future. The major work on the capitalized earnings approach, for example was contributed by Dublin and Lotka, demographers and actuaries, who also traced the history of thought on the economic value of a human life through the works of Sir William Petty, Adam Smith, William Farr, E. Engel, Irving Fisher, J. M. Clark and others.[1] According to this approach, the economic value of an individual's life is measured by the present value of his expected future earnings. However, this approach and other concepts employed for evaluating the loss or saving of life are unsatisfactory, because they are inconsistent with the Pareto principle. Mishan has indicated the inadequacies of the existing methods used and has developed a more appropriate conceptual framework that is consistent with economic theory.[2]

Studies of the benefit incidence of public health expenditures by income class generally have used neither the large body of literature on public health benefits measured on the basis of productivity and other concepts nor the theoretical approach proposed by Mishan. In this chapter, previous studies concerned with the measurement of benefits generated by health services will be surveyed and evaluated. First, methods employed in studies concerned primarily with measuring the benefits generated by health services will be reviewed. The discussion will include an evaluation of these methods and a summary of the theoretically founded approach proposed by Mishan. Second, how public health benefits have been measured and imputed to income classes in previous fiscal incidence studies will be reviewed, and shortcomings of methodology will be discussed.

Approaches to the Measurement of Public Health Benefits

Evaluation of existing methods and concepts

Four conceptual methods employed to evaluate the loss or saving of life may be classified as the: (1) gross output approach or capitalized earnings approach, (2) net output approach, (3) insurance principle approach, and (4) social point of view approach. Each of these is discussed below.[3]

According to the gross output approach, the economic value of an individual's life is measured by the present value of his expected future earnings, as mentioned earlier. The loss of potential future earnings upon an individual's decease may be expressed as

$$L_1 = \sum_{t=\tau}^{\infty} Y_t \, P_\tau^t \, (1 + r)^{-(t - \tau)},$$

where Y_t represents the expected gross earnings or value added by the individual during the t th year, excluding income he may have received from ownership of nonhuman capital; P_τ^t represents the probability in the current or τ th year that he will be alive during the t th year; and r is the social rate of discount that is expected to prevail during the t th year. This method can only be rationalized if the introduction or rejection of an economic policy is based upon its contribution to net national product; however, the maximization of NNP cannot be accepted as the objective of economic policy.[4] Most writers appear to have had reservations about the validity of this concept, despite its frequent usage and have considered it as only part of the total sum. Schelling, for example, distinguished between the value of L_1 and the difficult question of determining the value of life itself. He states that "so many examinations of the worth of saving a life are concerned with the fraction of man's income that he in some way contributes, that there may be a presumption that the outside limit of the worth of saving his life is the entirety of his expected future earnings. In fact there is no reason to suppose that a man's future earnings, discounted in any pertinent fashion, bear any particular relation to what he would pay to reduce some likelihood of his own death."[5]

The net output approach focuses upon the losses to others as a result of an individual's decease. The present discounted value of these losses to others over time may be expressed as

$$L_2 = \sum_{t=\tau}^{\infty} P_\tau^t \, (Y_t - C_t) \, (1 + r),^{-(t-\tau)},$$

where C_t represents what is expected at time τ to be the individual's personal expenditure during the t th period. The policy implications of the net output approach are clearly unacceptable, as it suggests that society is benefited by the death of an individual whose L_2 is negative. It implies that the death of most retired people would provide net benefits for society and ignores the feelings of survivors.[6] Consequently, this approach has not been employed, although some writers have mentioned it.[7]

The insurance principle method uses the probability that an individual will be killed and the premium that he is willing to pay to to cover that risk in order to determine the value that he places on his life. This method, however, does not provide the information required, even if the implied assumptions were acceptable, as the amount of insurance that an individual applies for does not reflect the value he places upon his life but rather his concern for the welfare of his family and dependents.[8]

Finally, according to the "social point of view" approach, an implicit value of human life may be estimated by examining the decision which society takes, through the political process, on public expenditures which may involve a reduction or an increase in the number of deaths. The existence of this method should not, as Mishan points out, relieve the economist of the task of evaluating some aspect of a particular project on the basis of an economic criterion.[9] Assuming that political officeholders try to obtain the maximum number of votes from their constituents by implementing programs that reflect the attitudes of a majority of their constituents,[10] however, this method may be useful in quantifying Mishan's proposed theoretical approach to the evaluation of life and limb.

Mishan's Theoretical Approach to the Evaluation of Human Life

Summary of the analysis

Mishan argues that none of the methods discussed above is consistent with the basic rationale underlying cost-benefit analysis, namely the notion of a "potential" Pareto optimum.[11] In solving allocative problems, the objective is to increase society's satisfaction and to achieve this, the criterion of a Pareto improvement can serve as a guide in ranking alternative projects. If at least one individual is made better off and no one is made worse off, the improvement is a Pareto improvement. A potential Pareto improvement is an alternative criterion of social gain according to which the net gains "can" be distributed in such a way that at least one individual is made better off while no one is made worse off. For example, a given investment project is likely to make some individuals better off and others worse off, when all economic effects are considered. If the project were to make a particular individual better off, the extent of his improvement is measured by a compensating variation, defined as the maximum sum, prefixed by a positive sign, that he would be willing to pay rather than do without the project. On the other hand, if the project were to reduce his welfare, the compensating variation would be the minimum sum, prefixed by a negative sign, that he would be willing to accept in order to tolerate the project. If the sum of all compensating variations for all individuals concerned is positive, benefits would exceed costs, and there would be a potential Pareto improvement through the introduction of the project.

If we are to be consistent with the criterion of a potential Pareto improvement, therefore, an individual's life should be valued by the minimum amount that he is willing to accept in exchange for surrendering it. Ordinarily, however, no individual may be expected to accept any sum of money, regardless of size, as a compensation for the loss of his life. Furthermore, it is highly unlikely that a project that entailed the certain death of any specific individual or group of individuals would be undertaken, regardless of the amount by which benefits exceed costs, calculated without taking these fatalities into account. Finally, when a particular project is introduced we can predict only that a given number of fatalities or injuries are likely to occur as a result of the project but we cannot indicate the specific individual or individuals to whom this will happen. For these reasons, therefore, Mishan argues that it is necessary to subtract from benefits the sums required to compensate each individual in the community for the "additional risk" which he faces as a result of the project, assuming universal risk aversion, rather than the amounts required to compensate specific individuals for certain death.[12]

Mishan's analysis is concerned primarily with the individual's response to a change in risk, rather than with a change in a statistical risk, as such. His analysis depends upon acceptance of the idea that the subjective preferences which people have for something must be taken into consideration. The amount of a collective good or "bad" is fixed for each individual, and his subjective preference for it determines his compensating variation (CV), which is the price that he is willing to pay or accept for it. An investment project may affect the welfare of each member of a community in a number of ways, such as by creating or eliminating employment, by making the development of commercial trade feasible, or by increasing the risk of death, and the latter needs to be included among economic effects.

Mishan considers the treatment of four types of risk: voluntarily and involuntarily assumed direct or physical risks and the financial and psychic aspects of indirect or derivative risks. In order to simplify the exposition of the analysis, Mishan restricts it to investments resulting in increased risk of death, but he also briefly indicates the symmetrical application of the same framework to the analysis of projects which reduce the risk of death and/or reduce the risk of injury or disease. His discussion of each of these risks is outlined in Figure 7 and summarized below. First, no special allowance need be made in project evaluation using cost-benefit analysis for "voluntarily" assumed additional risks of loss of life (R^1) as a result of a project.[13] To the extent that each individual evaluates such risks as a compensating variation, benefits are estimated net of these risks. The benefits are the maximum sums that individuals are willing to pay for the service while fully aware of the additional risks that would have to be assumed. The degree of risk that a given individual would assume voluntarily may be increased as the number of other individuals taking advantage of a given facility, such as a new highway, increases. These additional risks are "external diseconomies internal to the industry" and the individual may avoid them by not using the facility.

Economic activities also impose involuntary risks upon the community as a whole, risks which cannot be avoided without incurring costs, and cost-benefit analyses do have to make special provision for these risks. Mishan regards these as "external diseconomies external to the industry" and separates them into three types: involuntarily assumed direct or physical risks (R^2),[14] involuntarily assumed financial risks (R^3),[15] and involuntarily assumed psychic risks (R^4),[16] although any one individual may be exposed to all three and might receive a single sum as compensation. The direct involuntary risk of death is imposed upon individuals when an industry pollutes the air causing an increase in the number of deaths from respiratory and heart diseases; this is the primary risk from this activity. In addition, there may be a secondary risk of loss of life to those who may be infected by the direct victims of the activity. An individual would need to be compensated, therefore, both for the direct voluntary risk to him, even if he were the only individual in the community, and for the risk of infection imposed upon him by others. Where there is a risk of infection by others, it is difficult to distinguish primary and secondary risk. Mishan does not appear to find any advantage in maintaining the distinction in these cases; both risks are covered by the compensatory sum required by each individual.

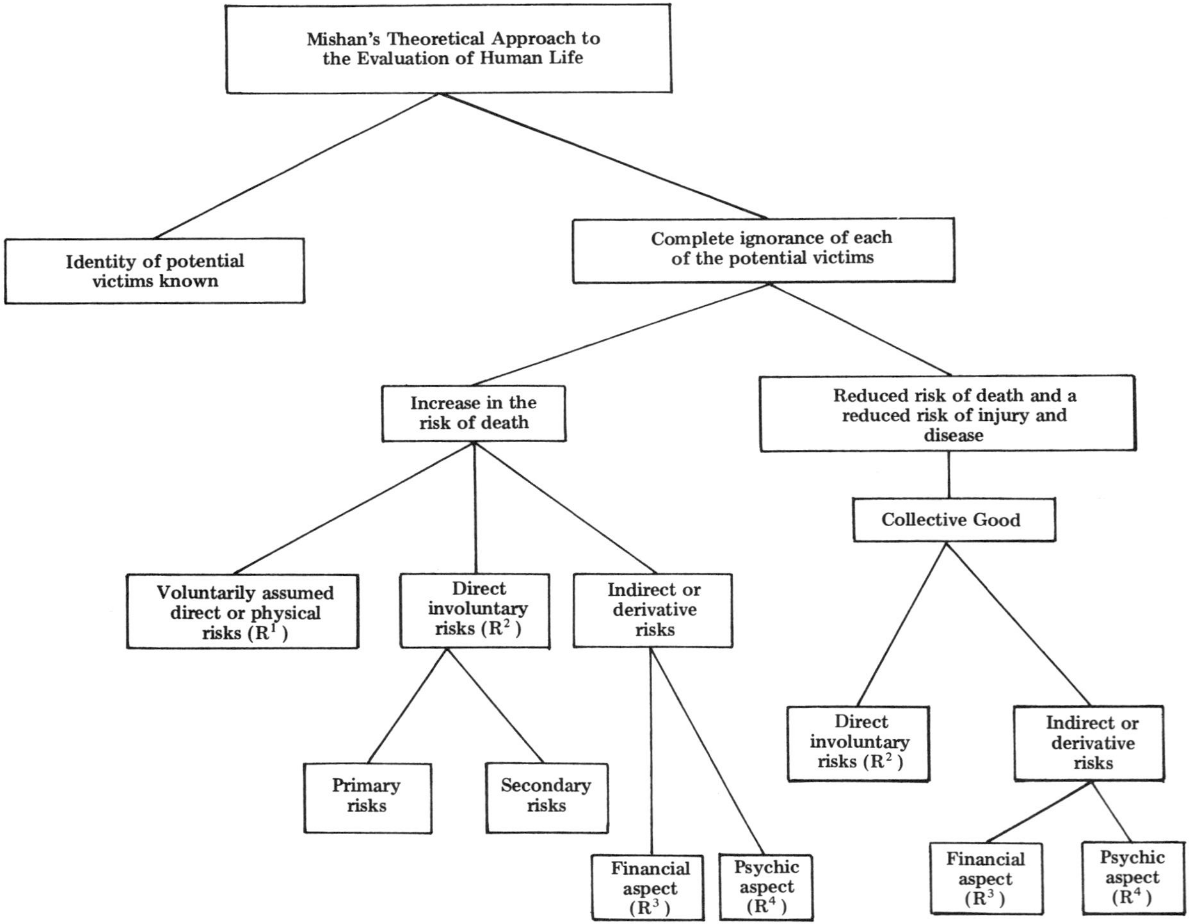

FIGURE 7: Mishan's Theoretical Approach to the Evaluation of Human Life: Analysis of risks associated with projects which increase or reduce the risk of death, injury or disease.

Each member of the community is liable to suffer additional concern as a result of the additional physical risks that a project imposes upon others. This additional concern may be separated into a financial aspect (R^3) and a psychic aspect (R^4). (See Figure 7.) A project may increase an individual's risk of experiencing a reduction in real income as a result of the death of another individual. The sum required to compensate him for this increased risk would therefore be positive. If, on the other hand, the individual's real income or financial position were improved by the death of another individual, he would be willing to pay a maximum sum for the greater risk of perhaps losing a dependent or inheriting an asset. The risk-compensating sum would therefore be positive. The total risk compensation for the community as a whole is obtained by aggregating the risk-compensating sums over all individuals. Depending upon whether the community as a whole expects its financial position to improve or deteriorate as a result of the deaths of others, this sum may be positive or negative.

Concern for the additional physical risks to others may also increase the risk of bereavement. This represents a loss of personal welfare for some individuals who require a compensatory sum to reconcile them to bearing the *additional* risk of losing family and friends; for the community as a whole, the risk compensating sum for increased risk of bereavement is obtained by aggregating the compensating sums for all the individuals and it carries a negative sign. This is the psychic aspect of indirect risks.

Analysis of public health projects designed to reduce the risk of death and disease, using Mishan's conceptual framework, is symmetrical with the above analysis of an expected increase in the risk of death as a result of a project, as illustrated in Figure 7.[17] In the above discussion, we have been concerned with external effects, which Mishan also refers to as collective goods and "bads," and in the case of public health projects we are concerned with a closely related concept, a collective good. The social benefits of purifying the air, for example, need to be compared to the costs of the preventive devices that are required.

Public health projects, regarding them as collective goods, involve only the three types of involuntary risks identified in Mishan's approach: (R^2), (R^3), and (R^4). As we are concerned with a collective good, there are no voluntarily assumed direct risks (R^1). The collective reduction of risk is the only good in question. Assuming universal risk aversion, a given individual is willing to pay up to some maximum amount in order to enjoy a reduction in the risk of death from involuntarily assuming physical risks associated with air pollution, the example mentioned above, including the primary risk to himself and secondary risk of infection from others afflicted with air pollution diseases. The total sum (R^2), is calculated by aggregating over all individuals and is positive. The risk of an individual being financially worse off or better off as a result of the death of another is also reduced with a reduced risk of death for all members of the community and the total risk-compensating sum (R^3) may be positive or negative, therefore. The fourth involuntary risk, the additional risk of suffering bereavement, also is reduced, and the total risk-compensating sum (R^4), is positive.

In conclusion, the basis for evaluating the benefits from a project that is expected to reduce the risk of death or suffering should be the aggregate of the maximum amounts that all individuals in a given region are "willing to pay" in order to enjoy the expected change in risk. Four components of the aggregate compensating variation for the community were identified, of which three were involuntary and one was voluntary. All of the voluntary risks are included in (R^1) and, since the benefits to an individual from the direct activity are already estimated net of this risk, it may be ignored. However, involuntary risks cannot be ignored. It might be conjectured, as Mishan does, that only one of these components, the involuntarily assumed direct or physical risk compensation, (R^2), may grow over time, as it depends upon the individual's preference to live; the financial risk compensation (R^3) may be expected to decline due to the growth of the welfare state and the development of a more equal distribution of real income, and the bereavement risk compensation (R^4) also may be expected to decline as a result of the development of an impersonal society and the weakening of family ties.[18] Mishan stresses that the compensating variation, or the maximum sum that an individual is "willing to pay" rather than forego an expected reduction in the risk of death, for example, is the only concept among existing alternative methods for measuring the loss or saving of life that is consistent with the Pareto principle, as it is applied in cost-benefit calculations.

Quantification of the social benefits or costs relating to a loss or saving of life

Empirically measuring the social benefits or costs relating to a loss or saving of life involves the same problems which were discussed in Chapter I. While we can directly measure the quantity of a particular good chosen collectively, measuring subjective valuations is not as straightforward. Mishan suggests that ". . . economists seriously concerned with coming to grips with the magnitudes may have to brave the disdain of their colleagues and consider the possibility that data yielded by surveys based on the questionnaire method are better than none, or better than data obtained by persisting with some of the current measures such as L_1 or L_2."[19] Another alternative, according to Mishan, would be to utilize contingency calculations. In his closing statement, he expresses what also should be the basic idea underlying current and future fiscal incidence studies: "in view of the existing quantomania, one may be forgiven for asserting that there is more to be said for rough estimates of the precise concept than precise estimates of economically irrelevant concepts. The caveat is more to be heeded in this case, bearing in mind that currently used and currently mooted measures of saving life or the loss of life—such as L_1, L_2, L_3, and L_4—have no conceptual affinity with the Pareto basis of cost-benefit analysis."[20]

Mishan's theoretical approach clearly is consistent with the "willingness-to-pay" method for imputing the benefits from public services across income classes, which was discussed in Chapter 1. The evaluation of the government program needs to be based upon the aggregate of maximal sums that all individuals in the region affected are willing to pay for the estimated reduction of the risk of death, an aggregate which may be divided into the three components, (R^2), (R^3), and (R^4), discussed above.

Measurement and Imputation of Public Health Benefits in Previous Fiscal Incidence Studies

In this section of the chapter, the methods employed to measure and distribute public health benefits by income class in previous fiscal incidence studies are reviewed and evaluated. In particular, it includes first, a brief survey of the procedures followed in eight previous studies, and second, an analysis of the issues regarding the methodologies employed.

Survey of Previous Studies

The eight studies discussed below were undertaken by the following authors and concerned the countries mentioned in brackets: (1) Gillespie (Canada),[21] (2) Gillespie (United States),[22] (3) Andic (Puerto Rico),[23] (4) Bhatia (Puerto Rico),[24] (5) Manrique (Colombia),[25] (6) Urrutia and de Sandoval (Colombia),[26] (7) Arellano (Chile),[27] and (8) Greene, Neenan and Scott (United States—all state and local governments in the Washington, D.C., Metropolitan area).[28] Of the studies listed, only that by Greene, Neenan and Scott computed benefits on a "willingness-to-pay" or "welfare" basis, namely, using the methodology discussed in Chapter 1; in all of the other studies, what Greene, Neenan, and Scott refer to as the "cost-of-services" approach, perhaps best exemplified by the two Gillespie studies cited, was employed.[29] Bhatia and others refer to the latter methodology as the "benefit" approach to allocating the benefits generated by government expenditures.[30] Bhatia distinguishes the benefit approach from what he refers to as the "money flow" approach, according to which:

> . . . the Government receipts are spent for the purchase of goods and services, such as from government employees, from sellers of goods to the Government, payments to bond holders, and to recipients of subsidy payments. This expenditure increases the money income of all such people. It creates a new pattern of income distribution if the recipients of benefits through government expenditures are different from those who financed the expenditures or if the proportion of benefits received from government expenditures is different from the proportion of burden arising from taxation. Under the money flow concept this redistribution takes place only with respect to those who are directly benefited by the Government expenditures or have to bear the tax burden directly.[31]

Under the money flow approach, for example, physicians and nurses are considered the recipients of expenditures on health services, whereas under the benefit approach, these expenditures would be allocated to those considered the ultimate beneficiaries of these expenditures. Bhatia regards the benefit concept as more meaningful in analyzing the distribution of benefits from government expenditures but, where feasible, he also uses the money flow concept. In his discussion of the money flow concept, Bhatia states that:

> . . . the money concept entails that the incomes of the employees of the Government would be zero if there had been no government programs. This assumption in a society where unemployment among people of the stature of government employees is insignificant is clearly untenable. The money flow concept, however, is justified wherever there are government expenditures consisting exclusively of transfer payments such as unemployment relief, old age pensions, agricultural subsidies, etc.[32]

Bhatia's discussion of the benefits generated under the money flow approach clearly refers to those benefits called source-of-income benefits under the willingness-to-pay approach. The appropriate theoretical definition of these benefits was discussed in Chapter 1.

Gillespie (Canada; United States)

As many fiscal incidence studies appear to have been modeled after Gillespie's studies of the incidence of taxes and public expenditures in Canada and the United States, several aspects of these two studies will be reviewed in some detail, including the (1) methodology chosen, (2) bases employed to allocate public health expenditures by income class, and the (3) definition of income. In both of these studies, Gillespie examined the incidence of all public outlays, health expenditures representing only one expenditure category.

Methodology

Gillespie considered two alternative approaches to analyzing the incidence of public expenditures.[33] Benefits could be measured by the "costs incurred on behalf of" various households. The average cost per family then would be distributed to those regarded as beneficiaries. Alternatively, benefits could be measured according to the valuation that each household places on the expenditures it receives. "Benefits received" would then be allocated to households in proportion to this distribution. Although Gillespie regards the second approach as preferable to the first, he considers the estimation problems almost impossible to overcome. It would require estimation of the revealed demand curves, or the underlying preferences, of each group of consumers for the services to be provided, and he considers this beyond the scope of his study. Gillespie, therefore, adopts the first approach, but he indicates that he does not consider this as serious a limitation as it might appear, as the two methods would coincide under certain conditions. He points out that if the benefits from a public good were received by a specific group of households and these households were to have similar income-earning or income-using characteristics, their demand schedules and, therefore, the prices which they would be willing to pay for the public good would be almost identical. If benefits were received by several groups, the above comments would apply if benefits could be clearly divided among these groups.

In determining the incidence of public expenditures, Gillespie treats the costs incurred by the government as an increase in the money income of those households on whose behalf they were made. However, he does not assume that these households would incur the expenditures. The procedure employed then was to identify beneficiary groups, calculate the average cost of providing the service to each of these groups, and determine the distribution of households by size classes of income within each group of beneficiaries. It was assumed that the value of total benefits received equaled total expenditures incurred, implying that the marginal cost of providing public services is constant (or that there is no consumers' surplus) and that public services are optimally supplied (or that there is no waste), as mentioned in Chapter 1. Gillespie considers it ". . . highly likely that the latter assumption will raise more objections than the former."[34] He points out, however, that the voting mechanism, though imperfect, permits households to eliminate zero-benefit expenditures or waste or at least to keep it to a minimum. Empirical estimation of the amount of waste in the provision of public goods was considered outside of the scope of these studies.

Bases employed to allocate public health expenditures by income class

Public health expenditures were classified under three categories: (1) public health, (2) hospital care, and (3) sanitation; then these were allocated to income classes according to the bases indicated in Table 2 below.

Expenditures on public health included programs aimed at preventing and treating communicable diseases, expenditures on general medical research, and some services provided free of charge to children of the poor who could not afford the cost. Gillespie argues that as a result of these services, the probability of contracting certain diseases is reduced, and if an individual has contracted a disease, the probability of his recovering is increased. He considers most of these services and expenditures on research as pure social goods which are available for consumption to all families in equal amounts, and he allocates expenditures for these services equally among all households.[35]

The procedures followed in allocating expenditures for hospital care in each study need to be explained separately. In the Canadian study, expenditures on hospital care included services extended under the Canadian Hospital Insurance Plan, which covers about ninety-five percent of the population. These expenditures were assumed to have been incurred on behalf of hospital patients and out-patients, on an emergency basis. To allocate these expenditures, Gillespie indicates that a distribution of hospital patients by income class, adjusted for the length of hospital stay, is required. However, data on hospital patients by income class were not available. Therefore, Gillespie allocated these expenditures under the assumption that patients were distributed randomly by income class.[36] The amount of hospital care provided below cost to the very poor was not known; this was assumed not to be significant enough to affect the final results and was ignored, therefore. In the study of the United States, expenditures on hospital care included services provided for indigents by general public hospitals and services provided by institutions for the mentally ill. Since these institutions provide services not only to the very poor but also to paying patients, expenditures on general hospitals were not entirely allocated to the lowest income bracket but were distributed across income classes on the basis of information regarding short-term hospital patients; data available on mental patients was used to distribute expenditures on public mental institutions.[37]

Expenditures on sanitation included expenditures for sewage disposal and waste removal. The benefits from these expenditures were assumed to accrue to the occupants of housing units, whether home owners or renters, and to the business community. In the study of Canadian expenditures, Gillespie argues that, in a perfectly competitive economy, the business component of these expenditures would be shifted forward to consumers. It was assumed that this component of sanitation expenditures was incurred on behalf of consumers. The ratio of the value of business property to the value of total property was used to determine the proportion of total sanitation expenditures allocable to the business sector. This amounted to thirty-three percent of sanitation expenditures, and these were distributed to income classes according to a series for total consumption expenditures. A distribution of home owners and renters by income class was used to allocate the remaining sixty-seven percent.[38] In allocating the costs of providing sewage control and other sanitation services in the United States, the industrial component was ignored, however. While a small portion of the costs incurred in order to treat industrial waste might have been allocable to industry, according to Gillespie, these costs could not be separated from those incurred on behalf of the occupants of housing units. A series representing a weighted average of owner-occupied and renter-occupied housing units was used to allocate all expenditures for sanitation.[39]

Definition of income

In order to analyze the effect of public expenditures on the distribution of income, expenditures are expressed as a percentage of

TABLE 2

Bases employed by Gillespie to Allocate Expenditures on Public Health, Hospital Care, and Sanitation By Income Class

I. *Public Health Expenditures in Canada by All Levels of Government in 1961*	*Bases Employed to Allocate Expenditures by Income Class*
A. Public Health	Allocated equally among all families and unattached individuals using a family distribution series.
B. Hospital Care	Assumed that patients were randomly distributed by income class.
C. Sanitation	Sanitation expenditures allocable to the business community were distributed using a series for total consumption expenditures; remaining costs were allocated to home owners and renters in proportion to the number of these in each income class.
II. *Public Health Expenditures in the United States by Federal, State, and Local Governments in 1960*	*Bases Employed to Allocate Expenditures by Income Class*
A. Public Health	Allocated equally among all families and unattached individuals using a family distribution series.
B. Hospital Care	
1. Expenditures on general hospitals for the care of indigents.	Allocation based upon a series concerning short-term hospital patients.
2. Expenditures on institutions for the mentally ill.	Allocation based upon rough data on mental patients.
C. Sanitation	A series representing a weighted average of owner-occupied and renter-occupied housing units was used to allocate all of these expenditures.

income. Gillespie employs two income concepts in his studies.[40] According to his "broad" income concept, income is defined to exclude the public sector or prior to the introduction of a public sector, and it consists of net money income plus nonmoney income (Y) and transfer payments (R), or Y + R. According to his "adjusted broad income" concept, income is defined to include the public sector, and it consists of the sum of: net money income and non-money income (Y), government expenditures on goods and services (B), and transfer payments (R), less tax payments (T), or Y + B + R - T.

Gillespie's results indicated that the incidence of public health and sanitation expenditures or the overall pattern of "effective" expenditure schedules was regressive or pro-poor in both studies, meaning that the expenditure rate decreased as income increased.[41]

Andic (Puerto Rico)

Most other benefit incidence studies are allocative exercises similar to those of Gillespie. Authors used whatever data were available and what were regarded as the most reasonable assumptions in order to allocate public health expenditures to income classes. Andic, for example, because of the lack of statistical information, used two alternative assumptions to allocate public health expenditures in Puerto Rico in 1955. From personal observation, he considered it reasonable to assume that low and middle income groups were the main beneficiaries of free hospitals, preventive medical and other health services provided freely or at very low prices. It appeared to him that upper income groups tended to use private hospitals, partially for prestige purposes. The lack of statistical information made it impossible for Andic to do more than roughly identify beneficiaries. The costs of providing these services were allocated first, equally to all families, and second, only to families with income below \$7,500.[42] The results obtained under the two assumptions varied little. (Andic presents a percentage distribution of total social expenditures combined, including expenditures for health, education, and housing for low income families, by income class, and these indicate that about three fourths of the benefits of these expenditures accrue to the three lowest income groups under both assumptions.) Expenditures appeared to favor lower income groups because of the relatively larger proportion of total families in these groups. Andic points out that while the assumptions may have biased the distribution of services received in favor of lower income groups, he does not believe that other allocative assumptions would have provided more satisfactory results. In fact, he suggests that they may have provided erroneous results. For example, if expenditures had been allocated either on the basis of the percentage distribution of personal income among income groups or on the basis of the relative expenditures on medical care by various income groups, he states that the distribution of benefits would have favored upper income groups. However, since these services are provided freely or at very low cost, expenditures for these services by lower income groups do not reflect the share of health services provided to them by the government. Despite the possible overestimation of benefits to lower income groups, therefore, Andic considers his assumptions to have been the most reasonable alternatives. Furthermore, the results are not interpreted as a definite measure of the benefits received but rather as indicating the government's intentions with respect to improving the distribution of income.

Bhatia (Puerto Rico)

Bhatia examined the incidence of public health expenditures in Puerto Rico on the distribution of personal income of families and unattached individuals. He classified total health expenditures in 1958 either as expenditures assumed to benefit the entire community or as expenditures assumed to benefit specific income groups within the community.[43] He found it difficult to classify health programs as either curative (infections or non-infections) or preventive, as some programs were both, and therefore decided to divide them into three categories: (1) programs beneficial to the entire community; these expenditures were allocated in proportion to the *aggregate income* of each income group; (2) programs which benefitted income groups up to $5,000; these costs and those included in category (3) were allocated to income groups in proportion to population or on a per capita basis; and (3) programs which only benefitted the income group below $2,000. In allocating the general benefit component in proportion to the income of families, Bhatia appears to have considered these expenditures as affecting the overall productivity of the economy as well as the distribution of income.[44] The effective benefit ratios or the ratios of benefits to family income were found to be progressive, meaning that the effective benefit ratio decreased with increases in income.[45] Bhatia's definition of terms progressive and regressive in analyzing the effective benefit ratio is the opposite of the conventional definition in tax incidence analysis; if the effective benefit ratio decreases (increases) as income increases, the incidence of benefits on the distribution of income is progressive (regressive). Gillespie, however, uses the terms progressive and regressive as they are employed in tax incidence analysis; if the effective benefit ratio decreases (increases) as income increases, the incidence of benefits on the distribution of income is regressive (progressive).

Manrique (Colombia)

As in studies by Gillespie and Bhatia, Manrique separated public health expenditures into two groups, those benefitting the community as a whole and those benefitting specific groups.[46] Public health expenditures in Colombia in 1966 were classified either as expenditures for environmental improvement, including campaigns to eradicate malaria and sanitary campaigns, or as outlays for hospitals and health centers. The former were regarded as social goods and allocated in proportion to the number of individuals in each income group. Manrique's per capita allocation of these expenditures, as in the studies by Gillespie, appears to indicate that he regards them as more related to the protection of life than to the protection of income or wealth. Manrique indicated that he regarded the services provided by public hospitals and health centers as generating positive externalities in the form of economic growth and an improved milieu, as a result of having a healthier population. In the calculations, however, the users of these facilities were considered the only direct beneficiaries. Poorer individuals in the rural areas of Colombia were assumed to share proportionately less in these expenditures than individuals living in urban areas because most hospitals and health centers are located in towns and cities and because of the low mobility of the rural poor and the poor system of communications. Therefore, only one-fourth of expenditures on health centers and hospitals was allocated to the rural population and the remainder to the urban population. These expenditures were then allocated to the six lowest income groups in each distribution, apparently in proportion to the number of individuals in each income group, although this is not stated specifically. Manrique estimates benefit to income ratios using a previous study of the Colombian income distribution by McLure based upon data for individuals, rather than households, in 1964.[47] He concludes that expenditures on public health are highly redistributive, with effective benefit rates decreasing sharply as the income level increases, but regards further public health expenditures as unlikely to significantly improve the situation of the rural poor. In addition to the problems concerning geographical location of hospital facilities and the dispersion of the rural poor and difficulties with communications, it was thought that cultural attitudes would prevent them from benefitting from such expenditures to any significant extent.

Urrutia and de Sandoval (Colombia)

Urrutia and de Sandoval, in their analysis of the incidence of public expenditures in Colombia on the distribution of gross personal income, allocated all public health expenditures in 1966 in accordance with the distribution by income class of the patients in a Bogotá hospital (Hospital San Juan de Dios).[48] This assumption was adopted because they lacked detailed data on both health expenditures and the socio-economic characteristics of the beneficiaries of these expenditures. Health expenditures included campaigns against communicable diseases and expenditures for hospitals and health centers. Expenditures on aqueducts and sewerage systems were analyzed as part of expenditures on development, which also included electrification, urban development, and housing, and allocated in accordance with the distribution of urban income. The authors regarded this as a realistic assumption, since upper income classes possess homes and durable goods that enable them to consume greater quantities of public services, including water, while the very poor, particularly in rural areas, dwell in houses lacking these facilities.[49] Urrutia and de Sandoval recognized the social good aspect of expenditures on sewerage and similar services. They suggest that these expenditures might have been allocated on a per capita basis to the urban population, since expenditures on sanitation benefit the community as a whole, and they indicate that the redistributive impact of these expenditures may have been underestimated by the allocative guide used. The expenditures allocated included only that portion of the costs of providing these services that is financed through the budgets of the three levels of government. Tariffs levied on consumers of these services were not within the scope of the analysis, but in Colombia this source of financing also is used to further distributional objectives; per unit charges for water and electricity consumed increase as the cadastral value of the consumer's property increases. The results indicated that expenditures on aqueducts and sewerage systems tended to benefit the upper part of the income distribution, but that expenditures on public health significantly contributed to improving the distribution of income. To estimate effective benefit ratios, the authors used the income distribution data estimated by McLure for 1964 and referred to above as having been used by Manrique, but they adjusted these data using the implicit

GDP deflator and growth rate of real GDP in order to estimate the distribution of income for Colombia in 1966.[50]

Arellano (Chile)

Arellano, in a study of the incidence of public health expenditures in Chile in 1969, allocated the costs incurred by the following public health institutions to assumed beneficiaries by income class, using the same methodology employed in the studies surveyed above: (1) The National Health Service (Servicio Nacional de Salud—SNS), which accounts for 80 percent of resources allocated for public health; (2) the National Medical Service for Employees (Servicio Médico Nacional de Empleados—SERMENA); (3) the Society for the Construction of Hospital Establishments (Sociedad Constructora de Establicimientos Hospitalarios—SCEH); (4) the Ministry of Health (Ministerio de Salud); and (5) Enterprises for Potable Water for Santiago and El Canelo (Empresas de Agua Potable de Santiago y El Canelo).[51] Expenditures on curative medical care provided by the SNS, for example, were allocated to assumed beneficiaries using survey data for 1968, while expenditures by the SNS on research and epidemiology were assumed to benefit all families equally. Expenditures on curative medical care provided by SERMENA, which is financed by monthly contributions of employees and contributions from the social security system, were allocated, net of estimated employee contributions by income level, to income classes in proportion to the distribution of employees by income class, as user data were not available. Investment expenditures by the SCEH were allocated by income class in accordance with income data available for hospital patients discharged from similar existing institutions, such as health posts. Expenditures by the Ministry of Public Health, which does not provide services directly, were allocated in accordance with a weighted average of the distribution of expenditures by income class of the SNS, SERMENA, and SCEH. Finally, expenditures by companies providing potable water to Santiago were allocated equally to all families living in Greater Santiago. The empirical results for the SNS, SCEH, and the Ministry of Public Health indicated that expenditures by these institutions favored lower income groups, while those of SERMENA and the water supply companies favored middle and upper income groups. Overall public health expenditures appeared to have a highly redistributive effect on the distribution of income as estimated expenditure to household income ratios decreased sharply as income increased.

Greene, Neenan, and Scott (All state local governments in the Washington, D.C., metropolitan area)

Greene, Neenan, and Scott analyzed the benefit incidence of public health expenditures by state and local governments in the Washington, D.C., metropolitan area in 1970 using the willingness-to-pay approach,[52] as mentioned earlier. Public health outlays included expenditures for community health services, such as tuberculosis control programs, the detection of hypertension, cancer, and glaucoma, and the provision of tetanus shots and pre-natal care; and expenditures for general and mental hospitals. As most of the community health services provided do not involve the externalities associated with the control of communicable diseases, it was assumed that the direct beneficiaries of these services receive: use-of-income, private benefits, if they have an income of $5,000 or more; in-kind transfers, if they have an income of less than $5,000. It was assumed that these in-kind transfers also provided public redistributive benefits to those with an income in excess of $5,000. The direct recipients of hospitalization were assigned use-of-income, private benefits, if they had an income of $5,000 or more; hospital services provided to those with less than $5,000 income were allocated to them as source-of-income transfers and those with higher income as use-of-income, public redistributive benefits. In allocating use-of-income benefits across income classes, it was assumed that the income elasticity of marginal utility is unitary, as stated in Chapter I. Total benefits from public health services, expressed as a percentage of the money income of households, were found to be "progressive" over all income classes, defined here to indicate that the percentage declined as income increased. At very high levels of income, however, the incidence was proportional and even slightly regressive at the very top of the income scale.

Although the authors regard the willingness-to-pay basis as theoretically superior, the distribution of benefits generated by public health services also was analyzed on a cost-of-service basis in part because these estimates could serve as a reference point in evaluating the results obtained using the willingness-to-pay approach and also because they have some analytical value. The results showed that the incidence of benefits from health services using this methodology is sharply progressive, that is, sharply pro-poor, over all income classes.[53]

Evaluation of Previous Studies

The studies surveyed above amply illustrate the conceptual, and statistical problems which bedevil the analysis of redistribution through public health expenditures. In the analysis in Chapter 1, it was shown that the benefit incidence of public health expenditures should be estimated in terms of individual utility. Value-in-exchange estimates for publicly provided health services, analogous to value in exchange of the private market, need to be established. To determine these, we must know citizen attitudes. However, since public services are not subject to a market test, such attitudes, or the "willingness-to-pay" for these services, must be discerned from information provided in attitude surveys and through the political process. Greene, Neenan, and Scott attempted to estimate the pattern of benefit incidence of public health expenditures on this basis. This methodology is employed in the empirical analysis in Chapter 4 of this study, although estimates also are provided on a cost-of-service basis, despite the limitations inherent in these estimates.

The following discussion focuses upon the major conceptual limitations of the cost-of-service methodology, some of which also apply to the willingness-to-pay methodology, in the light of the discussion in Chapter 1; several issues not mentioned previously also are discussed. The major conceptual problems with the cost-of-service methodology concern: (1) the choice of an appropriate counterfactual; (2) the equating of total benefits received with total costs incurred; (3) the identification of beneficiaries, particularly the failure to allow for public redistributive (use-of-income) benefits; (4) the evaluation of benefits on the basis of costs incurred on behalf of direct recipients, assuming constant cost per capita, rather than on the basis of individual utility; (5) the limitation of the analysis to short-run impact measures of incidence or first-round effects, that is, the failure to allow for general equilibrium effects over time; and (6) the implicit endowment of the *status quo* with normative value in estimating benefits by income class.

1. The Appropriate Operational Measure of Redistribution and the General Equilibrium Problem

In studies of the distributional effects of public expenditures, the observed incidence of public expenditures implicitly is compared with a hypothetical incidence pattern which is considered attractive as a normative benchmark. The only scholars who explicitly addressed themselves to the issue of what the appropriate counterfactual should be in analyzing the redistributive effects of government expenditures and taxation are Behrens and Smolensky.[54]

Behrens and Smolensky discuss what income redistribution studies should measure. They employ Musgrave's concept of "differential incidence," which was designed to address the general equilibrium problem.[55] According to Musgrave's procedure the gain or burden is measured by substituting the actual benefit or tax structure for a normative benefit or tax structure, involving the same total amount of expenditures or taxes; this procedure neutralizes the principal inflationary/deflationary effects of budgetary changes, although the general equilibrium problem is not fully resolved. For example, in studies involving differential tax incidence, the difference between the incidence of the present tax system and some normative tax system, such as a proportional income tax, is examined. In differential benefit incidence, an intuitively attractive normative incidence pattern is not available for comparison with the actual incidence pattern.

The redistribution that is achieved through government taxes and expenditures is defined by Behrens and Smolensky as the difference between a primary or benchmark distribution of income and a final distribution. They define the *final* distribution as "... the distribution of after-tax factor income plus transfers and benefits of all final government services. The benefits of general government services (which include any taxpayer benefits accruing from transfer programs) and recipient benefits of in-kind transfers are all valued at their marginal valuation to each individual as given by his demand curve for each service."[56] The primary distribution or counterfactual is defined in four possible ways. The meaning of each of these definitions and its important advantages and shortcomings are discussed below.

Gillespie or Zero Budget Counterfactual

The Gillespie or zero budget counterfactual is the primary distribution implicitly assumed in most studies of the distributional effects of public health and other government expenditures. The distribution of real income among households, given government expenditure policies, implicitly is compared with the distribution that would prevail in a no-government economy.[57] Equals and unequals are defined by the private market distribution of factor incomes. Behrens and Smolensky indicate that acceptance of the private market distribution appears to be based upon two principal rationales, a normative rationale that people should be ranked according to their marginal products and a taxonomic rationale that an overall measure of redistribution should include all effects of government.[58] They reject this counterfactual as inappropriate, since the government's function as a supplier of goods and services not provided efficiently by the private sector is ignored under this counterfactual. Factors may not be paid their marginal social products, if production or consumption externalities exist. Furthermore, the second rationale leads to an asymmetric treatment of the private and the public sector. If an activity is in the private sector, it is impounded in the counterfactual. However, if it is in the public sector, it enters the redistribution of income.[59] McLure points out that in a zero-government world, the "rules of the game" governing the operation of the economy might be different. There might, for example, be more or less monopolization thereby producing a different distribution of income.[60]

Lindahl I Counterfactual

Behrens and Smolensky propose a primary distribution that arises from a Lindahl equilibrium or the distribution that would prevail if only marginal benefit taxation were employed.[61] The activities of the private sector and the allocative activities of the public sector would bring about this distribution.

The authors found it necessary, in defining Lindahl redistribution, to distinguish between the allocative and the redistributive activities of the government. Two variants of the Lindahl distribution were proposed, which Behrens and Smolensky refer to as Lindahl I and Lindahl II counterfactuals. In the Lindahl I primary distribution, efficient transfers are viewed as an allocative activity. Donor and recipient benefits are assigned to the counterfactual and do not give rise to redistribution. Recipient benefits are not considered redistribution because the beneficiary is not merely receiving the benefits but also engaging in a productive activity. These transfers are treated as a service and considered part of the recipient's marginal product. The Lindahl I counterfactual differs from the zero-budget counterfactual, mainly because "... although benefits received by each individual are balanced by taxes paid, factor incomes may have been altered in going from zero government to the Lindahl equilibrium."[62] Redistribution relative to this counterfactual could arise through (1) deviations from the benefit principle in financing allocative expenditures, (2) non-efficient exhaustive expenditures, and (3) cash or in-kind transfers to some groups at the expense of others.[63]

This counterfactual appears to be conceptually defective. Since the primary distribution was defined as that which would arise if only benefit taxation were used, the treatment of Pareto-optimal or efficient transfers in Lindahl I is inconsistent with that definition. According to the Lindahl I counterfactual, these are not considered as a component of redistribution; they are enclosed in the counterfactual. Therefore, redistribution occurs only if redistribution is not Pareto-optimal. McLure objects to the counterfactual for this reason and also because under this counterfactual, the *net* redistribution attributable to the budget, after taking into consideration the benefits and costs of allocative expenditures financed by benefit taxation is calculated.[64] He favors retaining the additional information that would be provided by beginning with the zero-budget counterfactual, despite its shortcomings. Furthermore he objects to ignoring the impact of allocative activities of the government on the distribution of income, that is, ignoring expenditure incidence, by starting with a counterfactual that takes real factor income in the presence of these governmental activities as given.[65]

Lindahl II Counterfactual

In the Lindahl II variant of the Lindahl distribution, recipient benefits are removed from the primary distribution and consequently represent a source of redistribution in the final income distribution, while taxpayer benefits are treated as part of the counterfactual.[66] Therefore, true redistribution occurs only to the extent that transfers exceed what society requires in terms of transfers on the basis of interdependence of utility or Pareto-optimal transfers. McLure states that "to say that transfers benefit only those who pay for them, as alternative (b) Lindahl I does, is counter-intuitive, probably wrong, and not very helpful."[67] However, he considers the measurement of taxpayer benefits, as required in estimating the Lindahl II counterfactual, a difficult and controversial task.[68]

In their attempt to measure redistribution, Greene, Neenan, and Scott employ an approximation of the Lindahl II primary distribution. They are unable to use the precise Behrens and Smolensky definition of Lindahl II, as

> To estimate this counterfactual we would need to know the values that would place all citizens in a Lindahl equilibrium such that each citizen's marginal tax payment would equal the sum of his marginal nontransfer benefits from government services and his marginal donor benefits from transfer programs.[69]

They (1) assume that total expenditures equal the monetary value of total nontransfer and donor benefits; (2) estimate total nontransfer and donor benefits, evaluated at the margin, by income class; and (3) estimate the first component of distribution by taking the difference between nontransfer and donor benefits and taxes paid. They then (4) estimate the recipient benefits of Pareto transfers by income class; these constitute the second component of redistribution. Factor incomes are assumed to be the same in both the primary and the final distributions. Neenan points out that this assumption is less strong than that employed in many incidence studies, namely that factor incomes in the no-government case are the same as in the presence of government activities.[70]

In their evaluation of the Lindahl I and Lindahl II variants of Lindahl redistribution, Behrens and Smolensky express a preference for the former. They argue that "there seems to be no logical reason for excluding the payments for this particular activity from the primary distribution. An individual may incur a cost in receiving transfers (e.g., any associated stigma), as in other productive activities."[71]

Optimal Distribution or the Smolensky-Behrens Counterfactual

Finally, the authors proposed a primary distribution that is an optimal one. In the Smolensky-Behrens (S-B) counterfactual, allocative and redistributive activities of the government are based upon some ability-to-pay criterion in order to achieve an optimum. The difference between the actual fiscal treatment of individuals and the treatment that each would receive if the optimum distribution were achieved constitutes redistribution under this counterfactual. The authors state that ". . . any redistribution represents deviations from a specified optimum and can always be interpreted as detrimental,"[72] thereby turning around conventional analysis of the redistributive effects of government policies. The disadvantage of this counterfactual is that it requires that equals and unequals be identified and an explicit, normative judgment about vertical equity. In evaluating this counterfactual, McLure states that ". . . defining redistribution as failure to achieve an optimal distribution, . . . seems to serve no useful purpose, and to be nonoperational, in any case,"[73] since individuals cannot be expected to share the same views on what constitutes an optimal distribution. Behrens and Smolensky find this counterfactual appealing, however; they point out the growing support, among Thurow and others, for the inclusion of the issue of how to define an optimal distribution of income as a topic in economic analysis and the feeling that research is unnecessarily constrained by the failure to make explicit normative judgments about the optimal distribution of income.[74]

In conclusion, while Behrens and Smolensky prefer the Lindahl I or a combination of Lindahl I and the Optimal Distribution counterfactuals,[75] McLure favors the zero-budget counterfactual, but considers Lindahl II as "... probably the appropriate compromise."[76]

2. Equating Total Benefits Received With Total Costs Incurred

In all of the studies of the distributional effects of public health expenditures surveyed above, it was assumed that total benefits received equaled total costs incurred, assuming, as stated in Chapter 1, that public health services are optimally supplied and a constant marginal cost of provision. If the service is underprovided or overextended, total taxes collected will not equal total benefits. Furthermore, if average costs are rising (falling), the service may be optimally supplied, but total production costs will exceed (fall short of) total taxes collected. Unless a compelling case can be established for a suboptimal or superoptimal supply of health services, however, it appears reasonable to assume that the sum of the marginal rates of substitution of all households equals total taxes collected.

Benefits generated by investment expenditures generally also have been assumed to equal total expenditures incurred, in previous fiscal incidence studies, and authors have allocated them to the year in which the expenditures were incurred, ignoring the time dimension. This may be justified by assuming that benefits received from investment expenditures in previous years are approximated by current investment expenditures, but this assumption is incorrect when (a) the composition of investment is changing, and (b) investment is growing overtime. The assumption that total benefits equal total expenditures may be further criticized, as it ignores the likelihood that while most investments yield a positive return, some may yield a negative return. As the problem of how to treat investment expenditures in benefit incidence studies is unresolved, Greene, Neenan, and Scott focused exclusively on the incidence of current expenditures.[77] Snodgrass, on the other hand, estimated the incidence of consumption and investment expenditures separately and interpreted the latter estimates as useful ". . . to predict forthcoming changes in the distribution of public consumption benefits,"[78] similar to the assumption employed by Arellano in the study of public health services in Chile, discussed earlier.

3. Identification of Beneficiaries

In studies based upon the cost-of-service methodology, benefits were attributed solely to the direct recipients of the service in question. Assuming that the same cost was incurred for all recipients, costs were assumed to equal benefits generated and were attributed to recipients on a per capita basis. Allowances were not made for the external benefits of public health expenditures, particularly externalities arising from Pareto redistributive transfers. Free public health services for the poor, for example, generate Pareto-redistributive or donor benefits as well as benefits for donees. Only Greene, Neenan and Scott attempted to estimate these benefits as part of their willingness-to-pay methodology.

The provision of a sanitary water supply and sewage control generates another form of external benefit, referred to in Chapter 1 as public nonredistributive benefits. Urrutia and de Sandoval recognized the health benefits generated for the community as a whole by these expenditures, although they chose consumption as an allocation base, similar to Gillespie, who allocated expenditures on water supply to direct consumers. On the other hand, Manrique treated these services as pure public goods. In the empirical analysis contained in Chapter 4, it is assumed that a polluted water supply constitutes a central source of infection and the expenditures for the elimination of this provide public non-redistributive benefits to all income groups.

4. Evaluation of Benefits

Under the cost-of-service methodology, benefits are imputed on the basis of the costs incurred on behalf of direct recipients, rather than on the basis of the individual utility received from public health programs. Implicitly it is assumed that the marginal utility of income is constant across income classes. Aaron and McGuire have shown, as discussed in Chapter 1, that the imputation of benefits from pure public goods across income classes is highly sensitive to the specific utility function that is chosen, that is, to the values specified for the marginal utility of income. Maital, as mentioned in Chapter 1, proposed the following general functional form for the marginal utility of income:

$$MU(Y) = KY^{-\emptyset}$$

where $\emptyset$ represents the elasticity of marginal utility with respect to income, and he has argued in favor of a value of 1.5 for ϕ for the United States. Assuming a value of ϕ exceeding 1.0, implies that marginal utility declines more than proportionately with income; it implies that the monetary value of utility received by upper income groups will be substantially higher than when benefits are imputed under the assumption that the marginal utility of income is constant across income classes and that the monetary value of utilities received by lower income groups will be substantially lower. Maital's estimates of ϕ for the United States and other countries are based on the assumption of additively separable utility functions, implying that goods are neither complements nor substitutes, and his estimates were derived from private rather than public, sector data. For these reasons, as discussed in Chapter 1, his estimates may not be entirely accurate as a measure of the income elasticity of marginal utility for evaluating *public* services.

The marginal evaluation for public health services may depend on the size of the public health program itself and on the existence and size of private health programs and other public services.[79] Some private health expenditures such as those for hospital facilities, may substitute for public health expenditures, while other private and public health expenditures may complement each other, such as public expenditures on measures to control the incidence of disease, including expenditures on water supply and sanitation systems, and private expenditures on curative health care. A precise quantitative evaluation of public health services, or of particular public health services provided in Colombia, is not available. Therefore, benefit estimates in Chapter 4 are based upon what empirical data is available for the United States concerning citizen attitudes toward public programs, particularly welfare programs and other public programs of a redistributive nature. On the basis of these data, it is assumed that ϕ is unitary, as stated in Chapter 1.[80]

5. Limitation of the Analysis to Short-run, Impact Measures of Benefit Incidence

The redistribution through public health expenditures estimated in the studies discussed was based upon benefit and tax incidence estimates for a given year. The studies were limited to short-run, impact measures of incidence and no attempt was made to allow for general equilibrium effects. Future studies should, if possible, at least allow for qualitative estimates of general equilibrium effects. Even if redistribution can be accurately measured for a given year and expenditure and tax policies for that year are maintained, we cannot be certain that the estimated effects will continue to be sustained over time.

6. Endowment of the Status Quo with Normative Value

The Greene, Neenan, and Scott study as well as the other studies discussed are based upon the strong assumption that the utilities of individuals are derived from existing patterns of income, wealth, and talent. The status quo thus is implicitly endowed with normative value. This question needs to be addressed before any judgment regarding the social optimality of public activities can be reached. Benefit and tax-incidence studies, at most, permit us to infer estimates of welfare changes at the margin.[81]

Summary

The discussion of this chapter permitted us to see how health service benefits have been treated first, in studies concerned only with the measurement of benefits generated by health expenditures, and second, in empirical analyses of the distributional effects of public health expenditures across income classes.

From the analysis by Mishan, summarized in this chapter, we can conclude that the benefits generated by public health services should be measured by a compensating variation or the maximum amount that an individual would be "willing to pay" rather than do without the program, and this sum would have a positive sign. If an individual expected to be worse off as a result of a given project, the compensating variation would be the minimum sum that he would be willing to accept in order to tolerate the project, and this sum would have a negative sign. Finally, if the sum of compensating variations for all individuals concerned is positive, benefits exceed costs, and there would be a potential Pareto improvement as a result of the project. Other methods employed to evaluate the benefits generated by health services, such as the gross output or capitalized earnings approach, are inconsistent with the notion of a potential Pareto optimum, which is the basic rationale underlying cost-benefit analysis.

To summarize, Mishan is stating that the benefits from public health services need to be measured on the basis of a willingness-to-pay evaluation of government services as outlined by Dupuit in 1844. (See Chapter 1, p. 37.) The utility of the health service to the consumer is the maximum sacrifice that he would be willing to make in order to obtain it.

Mishan refines the analysis by systematically developing an idea advanced earlier by Schelling, namely that individuals are compensated only for the "additional risk" that a project may entail, as no sum of money may be expected to compensate for certain death; in the case of public health projects, an individual may be willing to pay some maximum amount in order to enjoy a reduction in the risk of death from involuntarily assumed physical risks, the risk of being financially worse off due to the death of another, and the risk of suffering bereavement.

In concluding, Mishan suggests that economists should endure the scorn of their colleagues and use survey data to measure subjective valuations empirically. He indicates that imprecise estimates of precise concepts are preferable to precise estimates of irrelevant concepts. As mentioned in Chapter 1, Neenan employed voting and survey data to develop an index of the willingness to pay for public services in order to impute perceived benefits generated by public programs across income classes.

In the remainder of this chapter, the procedures employed in eight empirical studies of the distributional effects of public health expenditures in various countries were discussed. In the study by Greene, Neenan, and Scott, benefits were measured on a willingness-to-pay basis, which was presented in Chapter 1 as the appropriate methodology for examining fiscal incidence. Therefore, the discussion of the conceptual limitations of previous fiscal incidence studies referred primarily to the shortcomings of the "cost-of-service" methodology, which was employed in the other studies. These included: (1) the implicit assumption of a zero-budget counterfactual, (2) the assumption that total benefits received by taxpayers equalled both total taxes collected and the total cost of providing the service, (3) the failure to allow for certain benefits generated, particularly public nonredistributive benefits to taxpayers who are willing and able to finance redistributive programs, (4) allocation of benefits to income classes on the basis of the costs incurred on behalf of assumed recipients, rather than on the basis of utility, and the implicit assumption that the marginal utility of income is constant across income classes, (5) limitation of the analysis to short run impact measures, and (6) the implicit endowment of the status quo with normative value.

The authors of the studies surveyed attempted, at least implicitly, to compare the distribution of income among households, given government budgetary policies, with what the distribution of income would be in the absence of government. *Redistribution* through taxes and expenditures is defined by Behrens and Smolensky as the difference between the primary distribution, which was the distribution of income determined by the private market in the studies discussed, and the final distribution of income, including after-tax factor income, transfers, and the benefits of final government services. Conceptually, the zero-budget primary distribution involves the following major problems: (1) if government expenditures were zero, the distribution of income would certainly be different from the present one, but we cannot determine how the distribution of income would be different, and (2) public and private production are treated asymmetrically, since an activity, such as the provision of health services, gives rise to redistribution if it is in the public sector, but is impounded in the counterfactual if it is in the private sector. Use of the zero budget counterfactual is a major conceptual shortcoming of fiscal incidence studies concerned with total government expenditures or taxes, particularly if these constitute a significant proportion of GDP, but is less important in studies concerned with smaller public expenditures, such as public health expenditures, which generally constitute a very small proportion of GDP, as the elimination of these would not significantly change the existing distribution of income.

Greene, Neenan, and Scott, as mentioned in this chapter, employ an approximation of the Lindahl II counterfactual, as defined by Behrens and Smolensky. Taxpayer benefits are included in the Lindahl II primary distribution but not donee benefits. Therefore, redistribution may arise through deviations from the benefit principle in financing allocative expenditures, including nontransfer expenditures and transfers required by donors on the basis of interdependence of utility; through recipient benefits of Pareto transfers; and through non-efficient exhaustive expenditures.

Identification of the various direct and indirect benefits generated by government expenditures and the need to impute benefits to income classes on the basis of utility, that is, issues (3) and (4), were discussed at length in Chapter 1 in the presentation of the willingness-to-pay methodology. As stated in this chapter, the proportion of benefits imputed to upper income groups could increase significantly, while that imputed to lower income groups could decrease significantly, in relation to what would be imputed to these groups under the cost-of-service methodology, depending upon the rate at which the marginal utility of income were assumed to decline.

Issues (2), (5), and (6), listed earlier, apply to both the cost-of-service and the willingness-to-pay methodologies. In all of the studies, it was implicitly or explicitly assumed that the supply of public health services is Pareto-optimal and that the marginal cost of providing these services is constant, in equating total benefits and total costs. Gillespie regarded the estimation of waste as outside of the scope of his studies, while Greene, Neenan, and Scott assume that the level of public services tends to be close to the social optimum. All of the authors focused exclusively on the estimation of short-run impact measures of the incidence of public health expenditures, without considering the likely general equilibrium effects over time. Finally, the last issue, concerning the derivation of the utilities of individuals from existing patterns of income, wealth and talent, thereby implicitly investing the status quo with normative value, has not been addressed in fiscal incidence studies.

NOTES AND REFERENCES

[1] See Selma J. Mushkin, "Health as an Investment," *Journal of Political Economy* 70 (October 1962): pp. 151-52.

[2] E. J. Mishan, "Evaluation of Life and Limb: A Theoretical Approach," *Journal of Political Economy* 79 (July/August 1971): pp. 687-705.

[3] For a discussion of each of these concepts see: *Ibid.*, pp. 687-91.

[4] *Ibid.*, p. 689.

[5] T. C. Shelling, "The Life You Save May Be Your Own," *Problems in Public Expenditure Analysis* edited by Samuel B. Chase, Jr. (Washington, D. C.: The Bookings Institution, 1968), p. 149.

[6] Mishan, "Evaluation of Life and Limb," *op. cit.*, p. 690.

[7] The following studies mention this measure: E. Devons, *Essays in Economics* (London: Allen & Urwin, 1961), p. 107; and R. G. Ridker, *The Economic Costs of Air Pollution* (New York: Praeger, 1967), p. 36.

[8] Mishan, "Evaluation of Life and Limb," *op. cit.* p. 691.

[9] *Ibid.*, p. 690.

[10] A number of studies have extended economic theory to political decisionmaking. Two important contributions to this literature are James M. Buchanan and Gordon Tullock, *The Calculus of Consent* (Ann Arbor: University of Michigan Press, 1965), and Anthony Downs, *An Economic Theory of Democracy* (New York: Harper & Row, 1957).

[11] Mishan, "Evaluation of Life and Limb," *op. cit.*, pp. 691-92.

[12] *Ibid.*, p. 694; see also Schelling, "The Life You Save May Be Your Own,", *op. cit.*, p. 142.

[13] Mishan, "Evaluation of Life and Limb," *op. cit.*, pp. 697-98.

[14] *Ibid.*, pp. 698-99.

[15] *Ibid.*, pp. 699-700.

[16] *Ibid.*, pp. 700-701.

[17] *Ibid.*, pp. 701-702.

[18] *Ibid.*, p. 704.

[19] *Ibid.*, p. 705.

[20] *Ibid.*

[21] W. Irwin Gillespie, *The Incidence of Taxes and Public Expenditures in the Canadian Economy* (Ottawa, Canada: Queen's Printer, 1966.)

[22] W. Irwin Gillespie, "Effect of Public Expenditures on the Distribution of Income: An Empirical Investigation," in *Essays in Fiscal Federalism* edited by Richard A. Musgrave (Washington, D. C.: The Brookings Institution, 1965), pp. 122-86.

[23] Fuat M. Andic, *Distribution of Family Incomes in Puerto Rico: A Case Study of the Impact of Economic Development on Income Distribution* (Puerto Rico: Institute of Caribbean Studies, University of Puerto Rico, 1964).

[24] Mohinder S. Bhatia, *Redistribution of Income Through the Fiscal System of Puerto Rico* (Puerto Rico: Puerto Rico Planning Board, 1960.

[25] Rodrigo Manrique, "The Incidence of Public Expenditures in Colombia" (Master's thesis, Vanderbilt University, 1972). (Xeroxed.)

[26] Miguel M. Urrutia and Clara E. de Sandoval, "Politica Fiscal y Distribucion del Ingreso en Colombia," *Revista del Banco de la República (Bogotá) 44 (*July 1971): 1072-87.

[27] Jose Pablo Arellano M., "El Gasto Publico en Salud y la Distribucion del Ingreso," Estudios de Planificación, Universidad Catolica de Chile, Documento No. 41 (October 1974). (Mimeographed.)

[28] Greene, Neenan, and Scott, *Fiscal Interactions, op. cit.*

[29] *Ibid.*, and The Urban Institute, "Unscrambling Metropolitan Fiscal Flows," *Search: A Report from the Urban Institute* 4 (January-April 1974): 3-8. De Wulf also is referring to what Greene, Neenan, and Scott call the "willingness-to-pay" basis for computing benefits when he discusses what he calls the "behavioral" approach. He considers this method ". . . highly relevant although extremely difficult and largely unexplored." See Luc De Wulf, "Fiscal Incidence Studies in Developing Countries: Survey and Critique," IMF *Staff Papers* 22 (March 1975): 79.

[30] Bhatia, *Redistribution of Income Through the Fiscal System of Puerto Rico*, *op. cit.*, p. 25.

[31] *Ibid.*, pp. 25-26.

[32] *Ibid.*, p. 26.

[33] Gillespie, *The Incidence of Taxes and Public Expenditures in the Canadian Economy*, *op. cit.*, pp. 88-91.

[34] *Ibid.*, p. 92.

[35] *Ibid.*, pp. 110-12; and Gillespie, "Effect of Public Expenditures," *op. cit.*, p. 148.

[36] *Idem, The Incidence of Taxes and Public Expenditures in the Canadian Economy*, pp. 112-113.

[37] *Idem*, "Effect of Public Expenditures," pp. 148-149.

[38] *Idem, The Incidence of Taxes and Public Expenditures in the Canadian Economy*, p. 114.

[39] *Idem*, "Effect of Public Expenditures on the Distribution of Income," p. 149.

[40] *Ibid.*, pp. 126-27; and *Idem, The Incidence of Taxes and Public Expenditures in the Canadian Economy*, pp. 6-11.

[41] *Idem, The Incidence of Taxes and Public Expenditures in the Canadian Economy*, p. 143; and *Idem*, "Effect of Public Expenditures on the Distribution of Income," pp. 138-39, 141-42.

[42] Andic, *op. cit.*, pp. 131-33.

[43] Bhatia, *Redistribution of Income, op. cit.*, pp. 45-46.

[44] De Wulf, "Fiscal Incidence Studies in Developing Countries," *op. cit.*, p. 26.

[45] Bhatia, *Redistribution of Income, op. cit.*, p. 33.

[46] Manrique, "The Incidence of Public Expenditures in Colombia," *op. cit.*, pp. 67-70.

[47] *Ibid.*, pp. 45-46; and Musgrave and Gilliis, *Fiscal Reform for Colombia, op. cit.*, pp. 239-52.

[48] Urrutia and de Sandoval, "Politica Fiscal y Distribución del Ingreso en Colombia," *op. cit.*, pp. 1078-79.

[49] *Ibid.*, pp. 1080-81.

[50] *Ibid.*, p. 1073.

[51] José Pablo Arellano M., "El Gasto Publico en Salud y la Distribución del Ingreso," *op. cit.*, pp. 1-43.

[52] Greene, Neenan, and Scott, *Fiscal Interactions, op. cit.*, pp. 78-79, 88-89.

[53] *Ibid.*, pp. 86-87.

[54] Jean Behrens and Eugene Smolensky, "Alternative Definitions of Income Redistribution," *Public Finance* 28 (1973): 315-32.

[55] See Appendix 1.

[56] Behrens and Smolensky, "Alternative Definitions of Income Redistribution," *op. cit.*, p. 317.

[57] See Gillespie, "Effect of Public Expenditures," *op. cit.*, pp. 123-24.

[58] Behrens and Smolensky, "Alternative Definitions of Income Redistribution," *op. cit.*, p. 320.

[59] *Ibid.*, pp. 320-21.

[60] McLure, "On the Theory and Methodology," *op. cit.*, pp. 14-15.

[61] Behrens and Smolensky, *op. cit.*, p. 318.

[62] *Ibid.*

[63] Behrens and Smolensky state that: "Although the Lindahl definition excludes the effects of allocative activities as an independent source of redistribution, the redistributive effects of *changes* in allocative expenditures induced by redistributive policies are included," in *Ibid.*, p. 324. (Emphasis theirs.)

[64] McLure, *op. cit.*, pp. 16-17.

[65] *Ibid.*

[66] Behrens and Smolensky, *op. cit.*, p. 319.

[67] McLure, *op. cit.*, p. 20.

[68] *Ibid.*, p. 18.

[69] William B. Neenan, "Income Redistribution," *op. cit.*, p. 7.

[70] *Ibid.*, p. 27.

[71] Behrens and Smolensky, *op. cit.*, p. 321.

[72] *Ibid.*, p. 322.

[73] McLure, *op. cit.*, p. 21.

[74] Behrens and Smolensky, *op. cit.*, pp. 322, 325.

[75] *Ibid.*, p. 323.

[76] McLure, *op. cit.*, p. 21.

[77] Greene, Neenan, and Scott, *op. cit.*, p. 4.

[78] Donald R. Snodgrass, "The Fiscal System as an Income Redistributor in West Malaysia," Economic Development Report No. 224, Development Research Group, Harvard University, Cambridge, 1972, p. 15. Cited by De Wulf, "Fiscal Incidence Studies in Developing Countries," *op. cit.*, p. 83.

[79] Neenan, "Income Redistribution," *op. cit.*, p. 14.

[80] See pp. 37-40.

[81] *Ibid.*, p. 25.

Chapter 3
THE PUBLIC HEALTH SECTOR IN COLOMBIA

Introduction

Health is probably both the single most important component of a standard of living and one of the most important determinants of that standard. The economic costs of ill-health include the loss of production attributable to disease and the expenditures for health services, which reflect the use of resources. Poor health status adversely affects the availability of labor for work due to absenteeism and mortality; the productivity of labor, due to reduced strength and stamina; and resource utilization, because calories are wasted when, for example, in the case of many parasitic diseases, nutrients are consumed by the parasites themselves, and when settlement of fertile land is restricted due to the prevalence of poor health conditions.[1] The Colombian authorities are aware of the obvious contribution that better health would make toward increasing both individual welfare and the productive capacity of a society by reducing the costs resulting from poor health and, in particular, of the effect that raising the health status of the poorer segments of the population could have on the distribution of income. Therefore, improving the health status of the general population is an important objective in Colombia's development strategy.

To stimulate economic development, it is thought that investment *per se* may not be sufficient—increasing the effective demand of lower income classes is also essential. In recent years, therefore, the Colombian authorities have attempted to increase employment directly through urban development, particularly the construction of low and middle income housing, through the promotion of labor-intensive export production, and through the stimulation of agricultural production and land redistribution; they also have attempted to increase effective aggregate demand, and, therefore, overall consumption, by achieving a more equitable distribution of income by both increasing the progressivity of the tax system and by broadening the scope of social services.[2]

By improving the income distribution, the authorities hope to systematically reduce one of the causes of under-development, namely, the dualistic nature of the economy. This dualism is characterized by the existence of wealthy and powerful families at the top of the income scale, with a high propensity to consume luxury and imported goods, and by the poor and unemployed, with a potentially large demand for Colombian-made goods, but with a very limited effective demand. By improving the distribution of income in order to broaden domestic demand, it is thought that more employment could be generated, and this would stimulate productive investment and yield the savings needed to finance that investment.[3]

Health expenditures are justified principally on the basis of their distributive effects.[4] Development goals, as in other countries, are no longer purely quantitative, but also include qualitative, welfare-oriented objectives. The authorities recognize the need to allocate resources for programs designed to directly improve the living standard of the poorer strata of the population, that is, programs which will help to achieve a broader distribution of the benefits of economic development. By reducing the gap in health status between the rich and the poor, public health services contribute to reducing disparities in the distribution of real income.

The purpose of this chapter is to review some of the great strides that have been made in the Colombian public health sector in recent years and to describe the functions of the most important institutions in that sector, particularly the Ministry of Public Health (Ministerio de Salud Publica) and the Colombian Social Security Institute (Instituto Colombiano de Seguros Sociales—ICSS).[5]

Historical Evolution of Health Policy

Colombian health services may be categorized into four groups, representing the initiatives and special interests from which they evolved.[6] One health service group originated in *Community Action* and was based upon the concept of eleemosynary and volunteer work advocated by charities and religious groups. These groups founded hospitals and other social welfare institutes and their philosophy was almost entirely curative. In 1913 *Government Action* began with the creation of a Superior Health Council, later renamed the National Directorate of Hygiene, which became the Ministry of Hygiene in 1938 and the Ministry of Public Health in 1953. Originally government programs were concerned with health protection and the eradication of communicable diseases through environmental control programs, such as the provision of potable water and sewerage systems, vaccination campaigns, and the isolation of groups constituting a hazard to the rest of the population. In Decree 3224 of 1963, however, this prevention and eradication function was broadened into a "health attention" concept, defined to include treatment for the sick, rehabilitation for the incapacitated, and protection for abandoned children and old people. A third health service group, *Welfare Insurance* plans for public and private workers, primarily emphasizes health recuperation. To a limited extent, this group also provides occupational and preventive health services. The fourth group, *Private Medical Practice*, provides ambulatory and institutional health services to the top 15 percent of the Colombian population which can afford these services.[7]

Health Systems in Colombia

Excluding private medical practice, there are three health systems in Colombia, which are characterized respectively as: official, mixed, and decentralized. Official institutions are financed wholly by central, departmental, or municipal government funds. Mixed institutions are financed by both government funds and other sources, such as donations and the sale of services to the community. Official and mixed institutions cover at least 70 percent of the Colombian population;[8] in 1970, this represented approximately 15 million people.[9] The decentralized system consists of social security institutions, such as the Colombian Social Security Institute (ICSS) and the various Cajas de Prevision Social. These provide health services to certain employee groups under the welfare insurance plans, mentioned earlier. They are self-administered and are financed primarily through employer and employee contributions, based upon established salary scales. These three systems have developed independently, with different institutional methods of operation and, as indicated, a variety of sources of financing. As a result, medical attention has been fragmented, and there has been a great diversification and duplication of installations. Hospitals, for example, frequently have been constructed as individual, self-sufficient institutions, without analyzing community needs. Consequently, hospital service has lacked stratification. Hospital beds have been poorly distributed, with too few in some areas and too many in others. During the period 1962-1972, only about 60 percent of total hospital capacity was utilized.[10]

Initiatives Taken During the 1960s

Major steps were taken during the 1960s both to improve the institutional structure of the public health sector and to provide more rational planning. In 1956, an initial ten-year health plan (1962-1971) began to be drafted with technical assistance from UNICEF, WHO, and PAHO. This effort revealed the severe limitations under which public health authorities were functioning, including the dispersion of responsibilities, the expenditure of funds without reference to priorities, patronage appointment of unqualified personnel, and the absence of reliable data on prevalent, major health problems. In response to this deficiency, the Colombian Association of Medical Faculties (Asociacion de Facultades de Medicina—ASCOFAME) conducted a national health survey of Colombia in 1965-1966, which has provided Colombian policy makers and planners with "... an extensive array of basic data on the health situation and the available health resources within the country."[11] The results of this survey were integrated into the National Ten-Year Health Plan covering the period 1968-1977, in which major programs were developed to reduce the most important causes of morbidity and mortality in Colombia. In 1967, a National Hospital Fund was established as part of the Ministry of Finance for the construction and equipment of hospitals throughout Colombia.

In 1969, a National Hospital Plan was prepared for the period 1970-1972, which includes criteria for the construction of hospitals at the various levels of medical attention, such as the university hospital, regional hospital, etc. as well as an analysis of institutional, human, and financial resources. The Fund is financed through the national budget, domestic and foreign loans, and through the sale of bonds to the Colombian Social Security Institute (ICSS). Furthermore, in 1969 an important policy document was prepared by the Ministry of Health, ASCOFAME, and the Special Health Projects Institute entitled "Levels of Medical Attention for a System of Regionalization in Colombia."[12] The document called for the establishment of a regionalized system of integrated health services, including contracts among university hospitals, sectional health services,[13] regional hospitals, local hospitals, and social security and welfare plan hospitals.

While these plans were being formulated, important national legislation was adopted authorizing the institutional and administrative reorganizations needed to implement them.[14] The Ministry of Health was strengthened and integrated policy lines were established by Decrees 1423 (1960) and 3224 (1963). As a result of

Decree 1499 (1966), regional (*departamento*) and local (*municipio*) health services became a decentralized function of the Ministry of Health. Finally, Decree 2470 of 1968 provided for the reorganization of the administrative structure of the Ministry of Health and the consolidation of its control at the apex of Colombia's public health system. Prior to this reorganization, the Ministry had been a relatively weak institution.

The Ministry of Public Health

Introduction

Within the public health sector, the Ministry of Health formulates health policy, approves and coordinates the proposed projects of all sector agancies that receive National Government funds, and through transfer payments from its budget, finances a sizeable part of the operations of these agencies. The Minister of Health presides over a Superior Health Council, including the directors of all principal agencies in the sector, which is charged with reviewing all programs for the health sector. The Boards of Directors of all major health agencies are also presided over by the Minister of Health. Outside of the public health sector, the Ministry works with other Ministries, such as the Ministries of Education and Agriculture, concerning health education programs and the implementation of massive campaigns against malaria and yellow fever in new colonization areas. Over the decade 1962-1971, when the major developments in the health sector discussed earlier occurred, expenditures of the Ministry of Health increased from 181.5 million pesos or 5.4 percent of the National Government's expenditures to 1,630.2 million pesos or 7.3 percent of its total expenditures.[15] As this study is concerned with Ministry of Health expenditures in fiscal 1970, the composition of these expenditures by function during that year is shown in Tables 2 and 3 below.

Health Promotion and Protection

Maternal/Child care

The single most important expenditure by the Ministry of Health in 1970 was that for maternal/child care, which accounted for 298.7 million pesos, or 23 percent of total expenditures. (See Table 3.) Strong priority is given to maternal/child care in Colombia, as women in child-bearing ages and children under the age of 15 constitute about 70 percent of the population and are the most susceptible to predominant health problems.[16] In 1967, children under 5 constituted only 17.7 percent of the total population, but contributed 46.6 percent to overall mortality.[17]

Other statistics concerning the five leading causes of hospital admissions and the ten leading causes of death in Colombia further illustrate the need to provide adequate medical services to this vulnerable part of the population.[18] Of the five leading causes of hospital admissions in Colombia, births, abortions and gastroenteritis and colitis of four weeks or more constitute the three most important, respectively. Gastroenteritis and colitis are particularly significant among infants and children under five, and of the ten leading causes of death in Colombia, gastroenteritis is the most important, followed by respiratory diseases, such as broncho-pneumonia and bronchitis. The high incidence of enteric diseases is attributed to poor nutrition, inadequate waste disposal, lack of access to potable water, and inadequate housing. These conditions also favor the high incidence of respiratory diseases, intestinal parasites, typhoid, and malaria.

The resources allocated to this program are channeled through the Ministry of Health to the Colombian Family Welfare Institute (Instituto Colombiano de Bienestar Familiar—ICBF), a decentralized agency, the establishment of which was provided for in Law 75 of 1968, and through the Medical Care Division of the Ministry of Health. The Ministry's objectives in regard to this program are to reduce morbidity and mortality among mothers and children under 15 years of age by improving child care and medical attention during pregnancy and during the partum and post-partum period and to supply family planning information. The ICBF conducts nutrition education and nutrition feeding programs for target populations, directs and administers orphans' and children's homes and family welfare pilot centers, attempts to improve family relations through educational programs and the provision of social services, and also protects children through legal actions against parents or guardians.

Sanitation programs

Colombia also has implemented successful, well designed programs in the field of sanitation, particularly in rural areas. Rural and urban sanitation programs combined accounted for 385.4 million pesos or 29 percent of the expenditures of the Ministry of Health in 1970.[19] (See Table 3.)

Sanitation programs constitute a major component of the strategy

TABLE 3

Ministry of Public Health: Total Expenditures by Function, 1970

	EXPENDITURES	
	(in millions of pesos)	(as percent of total)
TOTAL EXPENDITURES	1,308.7	100.0
CENTRAL ADMINISTRATION	4.1	0.3
General administration	(4.1)	(0.3)
SOCIAL SERVICES	29.7	2.3
Aged, orphans, etc.	(29.7)	(2.3)
PUBLIC HEALTH	974.9	74.5
Adminstration and technical services	(102.4)	(7.8)
Medical-hospital care	(281.4)	(21.5)
Maternal-child care	(298.7)	(22.9)
Environmental hygiene	(85.4)	(6.5)
Epidemiology	(174.1)	(13.3)
Other public health services	(32.9)	(2.5)
SANITARY SERVICES	300.0	22.9
Aqueducts and sewerage systems	(294.7)	(22.5)
Treatment of water	(1.3)	(0.1)
Latrines and septic tanks	(4.0)	(0.3)

Source: Contraloria General de la Republica de Colombia, *Informe Financiero de 1970* (Bogota, D.E.: Contraloria General de la Republica de Colombia, 1971), p. 135.

TABLE 4

Ministry of Public Health: Current and Investment Expenditures by Function, 1970

	EXPENDITURES	
	(in millions of pesos)	(as percent of total)
TOTAL EXPENDITURES	1,308.8	100.0
CURRENT EXPENDITURES	388.2	29.7
General administration	4.1	0.3
Social services (Aged, orphans, etc.)	29.7	2.3
Public health	354.4	27.1
Administration and technical services	(102.4)	(7.8)
Medical-hospital care	(163.3)	(12.5)
Environmental hygiene	(1.5)	(0.1)
Epidemiology	(61.8)	(4.7)
Other	(25.4)	(1.9)
INVESTMENT EXPENDITURES	920.6	70.3
Public health	624.7	47.7
Medical-hospital care	(118.1)	(9.0)
Maternal-child care	(298.7)	(22.8)
Environmental hygiene	(78.9)	(6.0)
Epidemiology	(112.3)	(8.6)
Other public health services	(16.7)	(1.3)
Sanitary services	296.0	22.6
Aqueducts and sewerage systems	(290.7)	(22.2)
Treatment of water	(1.3)	(0.1)
Water closets and septic tanks	(4.0)	(0.3)

Sources: Contraloria General de la Republica de Colombia, *Informe Financiero de 1970* (Bogota, D.E.: Contraloria General de la Republica de Colombia, 1971), pp. 134-35; Direccion General del Presupeuesto, *Presupuesto de Colombia: 1970* (Bogota, D.E.: Direccion General del Presupuesto, 1970), pp. 155-89, 551-69.

to improve health status in Colombia, as poor sanitation conditions have significantly contributed to high sickness and death rates. About half of transmittable diseases in Colombia are transmitted by water, and it has been estimated that 14 percent of deaths are caused by water-borne diseases.[20] The high rates of gastroenteritis are caused by bacteria transmitted through contaminated food and contaminated water, and by parasites, such as ascaridiasis and trichuriasis (transmitted through the mouth) and uncinariasis (transmitted through the skin), all of which are also associated with contaminated water and poor waste disposal, and to a lesser extent by viruses. Intestinal parasites may be eradicated by providing potable water and adequate waste disposal services, particularly in rural areas, where incidence rates are highest. In addition, hygienic habits in food preparation need to be taught and controls implemented over individuals who sell food or handle it in public eating places.

Rural sanitation

Basic rural sanitation is the responsibility of the National Institute of Special Health Programs (Instituto Nacional Para Programas Especiales de Salud — INPES), which provides potable water and sewage disposal systems in rural areas, that is, to communities with up to 2,500 inhabitants; these accounted for about 8 million people or two-fifths of the total population in 1971.[21] The activities of INPES are recorded in Table 2 as environmental hygiene (water supply in rural areas), treatment of water, and latrines and septic tanks. Decree 477 of 1968 provided for the establishment of the Institute as a public, decentralized entity. Its services are financed through transfer payments from the national budget, external loans, and community contributions. Prior to 1968, a program for basic rural sanitation had existed in the Ministry of Health. In addition to providing basic rural sanitation, INPES also provides services through its Special Research Division, which carries out studies in the health field, and through its Division of the National Health Laboratory, called "Samper Martinez," which produces the biologic products needed for massive vaccination campaigns in Colombia and markets these in other Latin American countries as well. Samper Martinez also carries out research and teaching activities.

The benefits of INPES' rural sanitation program may be regarded as extending beyond the expected significant impact on health due to disease eradication to the strengthening of socio-political development in Colombia. Community action constitutes an important aspect of the program; local groups request the project; help to construct it by contributing labor, material and economic resources; participate in its operation, maintenance, and administration; and amortize the investment expenditures. The execution of a project begins with an inventory by an INPES promoter at one of the 24 departmental sections of INPES. He examines the sanitary, economic, social, and cultural characteristics of the community which might have a bearing upon the project. The promoter may then establish contacts with local authorities and organized groups, and if these are sufficiently motivated, a contract is signed between the Community Action Group and INPES governing the project's construction, financing, and administration. INPES prepares topographic designs and construction plans, contracts a construction supervisor, and controls the progress of the work and the community's contribution. Upon completion, the project is turned over to a Board of Administration established for each project and consisting of three members, a representative of the Community Action Group of the local community, a representative of the users of the services, and a representative of INPES. The Board is charged with maintaining the project and amortizing its cost, and these Boards have proven to be highly effective. The local community generally contributes about 20 percent of the project's costs in the form of labor and economic resources.[22] Some of the investment costs may be covered by grants, and the rest, about 50 percent of costs, is financed through a ten to fifteen year loan carrying a 6 percent interest charge.[23]

INPES projects also generate other economic and social benefits.[24] For example, they have provided the basic services needed for the development of small industry, promoted the training of workers and plumbers, and eliminated time lost in transporting water. The INPES program, however, may also be viewed as strengthening the government's role as an integrative social force. Health may be considered among society's most deeply felt needs, and to the extent that government can provide the public services to satisfy this need, society may develop a positive attitude toward government. A program such as this may particularly favor political development as it is based on community action, as mentioned above, is usually the first genuine community project to be undertaken, and the experience thereby acquired frequently leads to further active community involvement in development.

Urban sanitation

Public services in Colombia's rapidly growing urban areas also have been inadequate, expecially in the supply of potable water and the removal of water borne wastes. In 1970, 294.7 million pesos, or 22.5 percent of expenditures of the Ministry of Health was allocated for urban sanitation projects. These funds were transferred through the Ministry of Health to the national agency responsible for water supply and sewerage projects in Colombia, the National Institute for Municipal Development (Instituto de Fomento Municipal—INSFOPAL), and to municipal public enterprises. Twenty-one of Colombia's cities, with a combined population of about 7.5 million in 1970, one-third of the total population, have their own municipal companies, which provide public services. INSFOPAL serves urban areas with more than 2,500 inhabitants, approximately 750 towns, accounting in 1971 for about 5.3 million people, or one-fourth of Colombia's population.[25] The institute was established in 1936 and functioned under the supervision of the Ministry of Public Works until 1968, when Decree 3178 provided for it to be placed under the supervision of the Ministry of Health. INSFOPAL prepares, constructs, operates, and maintains investment projects in the water supply and sewerage sector.

Urban sanitation projects form part of the government's strategy for channeling the growing urban migration to medium sized cities, rather than to major urban areas, by providing them with better public services. This should promote the development of these areas and alleviate the strain on public services in Colombia's major urban centers.

Epidemiology

In the area of health protection, Colombia, in recent years, has conducted massive vaccination campaigns against smallpox, tuberculosis, dipththeria, whooping cough, tetanus, polio and measles. These programs are well coordinated within the health sector. The Ministry of Health determines the areas and age groups to be vaccinated, INPES' Samper Martinez Laboratory prepares the vaccines, and the sectional health services carry out the actual vaccination and implementation.

Altitude and temperature conducive to malaria prevail in about 85 percent of Colombia. The National Service for the Eradication of Malaria (Servicio Nacional de Erradicacion de la Malaria—SEM) which is part of the Ministry of Health, conducts campaigns against malaria, yellow fever, yaws, and other diseases in these zones. These efforts are particularly important in new agricultural colonization areas. In 1970, about 13 percent of the Ministry of Health's expenditures, or 174 million pesos, was allocated for vaccination campaigns and direct campaigns against the other diseases mentioned. (See Table 3.)

Health Recuperation

Expenditures for medical-hospital care only represented about 21 percent of the total expenditures of the Ministry of Health in 1970, but these expenditures contribute to the financing of outpatient and hospital services covering about 70 percent of the population, as mentioned earlier. These services are provided by official and mixed institutions. In 1972, these institutions provided 40 percent of total medical consultations, and of the 1,184,863 persons hospitalized, 69 percent were hospitalized in official and mixed institutions.[26] The construction, completion, and the purchase of equipment for hospitals, health posts, and health centers accounted for 118.1 million of the 163.3 million allocated for medical-hospital care in 1970. (See Table 4.) Expenditures for the maintenance of these institutions, the formulation of health programs, and transfers to the National Cancer Institute to provide diagnosis and treatment services accounted for the rest. Many of the Ministry's programs, including those concerning medical attention, hospital construction, and massive vaccination campaigns, are carried out by the sectional health services. The sectional health services are connected with local and regional hospitals, including those formerly dependent upon charity funds.

The 1966 National Morbidity Census provided some information on the demand for medical services based on home interviews.[27] According to this survey, 387 per 1,000 felt ill during the two weeks before the interviews; of these only 88 had consultation.[28] Of the 88, 63 saw a physician, while the rest consulted pharmacists, nurses, midwives, dentists, or their families. The results of the study also showed that only 38 percent of the population received the 40,670,000 medical consultations which took place in 1965. This amounted to an average of 6.1 consultations per person in this group. The rest of the population, however, did not receive attention. Data was also collected for women between the ages of 15 and 54 and retrospective for 9 to 15 months.[29] Of the 867,000 pregnancies culminated during this period, 48 percent received the attention of a physician; in rural areas, only 31 percent of the pregnancies culminated received the attention of a physician. An estimated 745,000 of these pregnancies resulted in births, 34 percent of which were attended by physicians, 55 percent by midwives or nurses, and the rest by other individuals.

Other Expenditures

Administrative expenditures relating to public health services consist of the development of health plans for the sectional health services, the preparation of the national Health Plan, and the supervision and evaluation of the activities financed.

Finally, numerous welfare institutions known as "centros de beneficencia" also are financed partially through the Ministry's budget. These include old age homes, orphanages, child welfare centers, rehabilitation centers, dispensaries, nurseries, child care centers, and milk distribution centers.

The Colombian Social Security Institute

Introduction

The Colombian Social Security Institute, Instituto Colombiano de Seguros Sociales (ICSS), and similar welfare insurance organizations also account for a substantial share of public sector health expenditures.[30] ICSS is by far the most important of these in terms of financial resources and coverage. All private enterprises must enroll their employees in the system. As a result, about 35 percent of the employed urban labor force is insured by ICSS, the rest consisting mainly of public sector employees at the departmental, municipal, and national level, who have their own social security plans and self-employed individuals.[31] In 1971, ICSS covered 1,014,947 insured employees, including 16,608 retired employees,[32] whereas social security plans providing medical attention to public employees only covered 124,029 beneficiaries.[33] (Under the General Health and Maternity Insurance scheme, ICSS covered 943,483 insured employees and 374,521 dependents in 1971.)[34] Within the public sector, the revenues of ICSS are second in magnitude only to those of the Central Government, exceeding those of every other public enterprise and decentralized agency. These revenues are used not only to finance health services, but also are set aside as pension reserves and invested.

Insurance Programs and Administration

ICSS was founded with the enactment of Law 90 in 1946 as an agency with judicial independence and attached to the Ministry of Labor. This law marked the beginning of a comprehensive social security program, combining health, disability and retirement insurance. The plan consists of the following three programs: (1) general health and maternity insurance, introduced in 1949, (2) occupational illness and work insurance, introduced in 1965, and (3) invalidism, old age and death benefits, which began in 1967.[35] The basic provisions of each insurance program are outlined in Table 5, including a description of the benefits provided and how they are financed.

TABLE 5

Colombian Social Security Institute: Health, Disability and Retirement Insurance

I. *Insurance Programs*

A. *General Health and Maternity Insurance* (El Seguro Social Obligatorio de Enfermedad No Profesional y Maternidad—E.Y.M.), introduced in 1949.
B. *Occupational Illness and Work Insurance* (El Seguro Social Obligatorio de Accidentes de Trabajo y Enfermedades Profesionales—R.P.), introduced in 1965.
C. *Invalidism, Old Age, and Death Benefits* (El Seguro Social Obligatorio de Invalidez, Vejez y Muerte—I.V.M.), introduced in 1967.

II. *Definition of Illnesses Relating to Each Program*

A. *General Health and Maternity Insurance*
Illnesses that are not attributable solely to the job or profession of the insured or that are not especially tied to his work, such as sinus, influenza, or cardiac problems.
B. *Occupational Illness and Work Insurance*
Illnesses necessarily tied to the occupation of the insured, as, for example, silicosis among miners.
C. *Invalidism, Old Age, and Death Benefits*
The same as for General Health and Maternity Insurance.

III. *Economic Assistance in Cases of Illness*

A. *Subsidies*
Paid only during the recuperative period and when the incapacity is temporary, that is, not permanent.
1. *General Health and Maternity Insurance*
Illnesses unrelated to job or profession: the patient receives two thirds of his base salary as of the fourth day of his illness; the subsidy is paid for a period of up to 180 days.

2. *Occupational Illness and Work Insurance*

   Illnesses related to job or profession: the patient receives 100 percent of his base salary as of the first day of his illness; he may receive the subsidy for an indefinite period that is, until he is cured or it has been determined that the injury is incurable.

3. *Invalidism, Old Age, and Death Benefits*

   The patient may receive subsidies in substitution for his salary for a period of up to 180 days under the General Health and Maternity Insurance scheme, when the incapacity is temporary. These subsidies equal two-thirds of his base salary. If he is not cured within this period of time, he may receive a Disability Pension under the Invalidism, Old Age, and Death Benefits scheme amounting to four-fifths of his base salary.

B. *Pensions*

1. *Occupational Illness and Work Insurance*

   a) *Permanent Partial Incapacity* (Invalidez Permanente Parcial)

   The disability is permanent, but capacity to work has not been totally eliminated.

   The pension is proportional to that which the insured would have been entitled to in the case of total permanent incapacity and in accordance with the percentage valuation of his incapacity. For example, for an individual who has lost 30 percent of his capacity to work and whose base salary is 1,000 pesos, the pension in the case of total permanent incapacity would be 600 pesos (60 percent of his base salary). The pension in the case of Permanent Partial Incapacity would be 180 pesos (30 percent of 600 pesos). If his loss of capacity to work lies between 5 percent and 20 percent, he is paid an indemnity calculated as above, and equal to 36 monthly payments.

   b) *Permanent Total Incapacity* (Incapacidad Permanente Total)

   Diminished capacity to carry out one's occupation or profession, as in the case of the loss of a hand by a typist.

   The monthly pension is equivalent to 60 percent of the monthly base salary.

   c) *Permanent Absolute Incapacity* (Incapacidad Permanente Total)

   Incapacity to carry out any work activity or profession, as, for example, due to the loss of both hands.

The monthly pension is equivalent to 70 percent of the monthly base salary.

d) *Great Incapacity* (La Gran Invalidez)

The patient needs assistance in order to carry out the elementary activities of life as, for example, an individual who is unable to move himself alone or eat alone.

The monthly pension is equivalent to 85 percent of the monthly base salary.

e) *Death*

A lifelong pension is paid to the widow equivalent to 23 percent of the decedent's base salary. Pensions are also paid for every child until he reaches the age of 18, if he is a student; the pension is equal to 15 percent of the decedent's base salary.

2. *Invalidism, Old Age, and Death Benefits*

a) *Invalidism and Old Age*

The pension consists of 45 percent of the base salary plus 14 percent of the minimum pension in force for the wife and 7 percent of the same pension for each child.

In the cases of both death and invalidism, in order to receive a pension, the insured must have contributed for a minimum of 150 weeks, and 75 of these must have been during the three previous years. In the case of old age, the insured must have contributed for 500 weeks, the last of which must have been paid within the ten years immediately preceding the date on which the insured reaches the age of 60, in the case of men, of 55 in the case of women.

b) *Death*

A pension is paid to the widow and financial support is provided for the children. These are determined as follows: first, the pension that would have been received by the decedent in the case of old age or invalidism is determined; second, 50 percent of this amount is allowed for the widow and 20 percent for each child, but the total amount may not exceed 100 percent of the pension that is paid in the case of invalidism.

IV. *Maternity: Economic and Medical Assistance Accorded to Beneficiaries Under the General Health and Maternity Insurance Scheme*

A. *Insured Female Employees*

1. *Medical Care*

Monthly consultations during pregnancy; hospitalization;

surgery, if necessary; medical care during the partum and post partum periods.

2. *Economic Assistance*

A financial subsidy is paid equal to 100 percent of the insured patient's base salary for 56 days. Originally, this had to be taken 28 days before delivery and 28 days after, but now the entire 56 days may be taken after the delivery.

B. *Benefits for the Infant*

Total medical, pharmaceutical, hospital, and surgical care during the first 12 months of life.

C. *Wife or Common Law Wife (Compañera) of an Insured Employee*

Entitled to complete medical care but not financial subsidies.

V. *Financing of the Three Insurance Programs*

A. *General Health and Maternity Insurance and Invalidism, Old Age, and Death Benefits*

Financing is shared between the employer and the employee; it is distributed as follows: one-third is paid by the employee, two-thirds by the employer. Contributions are made according to a different scale of fixed absolute amounts for each program. In the case of General Health and Maternity Insurance, the employer contributes an amount equal to about 4.7 percent of the employee's base salary and the employee contributes an amount equal to about 2.3 percent of his base salary.[36] In the case of Invalidism, Old Age and Death Benefits, the employer contributes an amount equal to 3.0 percent of the employee's base salary, and the employee contributes an amount equal to 1.5 percent of his base salary.[37]

B. *Occupational Illness and Work Insurance*

Contributions are entirely paid by the employer and are based not only on the amount of the base salary but also on the type of activity carried out in the respective enterprise, taking into account the degree of danger associated with each activity. For this purpose, risk categories were designed.

VI. *Distribution and Management of Revenues Between National and Local Administrations*

A. *Occupational Illness and Work Insurance and Invalidism, Old Age, and Death Benefits*

Contributions are sent to the Central Office, as these are managed directly by the Institute at the national level.

B. *General Health and Maternity Insurance*

Contributions remain in Local Offices (Oficinas Locales) and Local Branches (Cajas Seccionales) where they are collected and expended.

The budgets of the Local Branches need not be approved by the Central Office, but Local Offices need such approval.

The financial resources of the General Health and Maternity Insurance scheme have been supplemented through financial payments out of the Solidarity Fund (Fondo de Solidaridad); this fund consists of limited transfers received from the other insurance programs, that is, from Occupational Illness and Work Insurance and from Invalidism, Old Age, and Death Benefits, and of transfers received from the Central Government.

These different programs are administered at the national level by a Board of Directors consisting of the Minister of Labor and Social Security (or his Vice Minister), who presides over the Board, the Minister of Health (or his Vice Minister), and an employers' representative, a workers' representative, and a representative of the medical profession. The president of Colombia selects the non-governmental representatives on the Board and also appoints a General Manager for the Institute. At the regional level, these programs are administered by Sectional Branches (Cajas Seccionales) and Sectional Offices (Oficinas Seccionales), the former having more administrative and financial autonomy than the latter.

Health Services

Objectives

Fundamentally, the objectives of the system are to end incapacity to work due to illness by providing complete medical, surgical, pharmaceutical, hospital and dental care; provide financial assistance during a period when work is interrupted as a result of illness, accidents, incapacity, old age, or death; and prevent loss of capacity to work as a result of illness or accidents by promoting professional reeducation.[38]

Distribution of expenditures on health services

In 1970, total health expenditures by ICSS for the beneficiaries of the three insurance schemes mentioned amounted to 887.8 million pesos, or about 55 percent of total current revenue.[39] As shown in Table 6, the single most important expenditure item was hospitalization, including surgery and obstetrics; it accounted for 254.9 million pesos, or 28.7 percent of the total. Expenditures for medical and dental consultations, which constituted the second largest expenditure item, amounted to 185.5 million pesos, or 20.9 percent of total expenditures. As part of the General Health and Maternity Insurance scheme, subsidies were paid to patients temporarily unable to work because of illness and in maternity cases; as indicated in Table 6; these only involved 55.4 million pesos, or 6.2 percent of expenditures. Subsidies are related to an individual's base salary (*salario de base*), and authorization to be paid subsidies must be obtained from a physician. The Institute had grouped all affiliated individuals by income brackets and has set a base salary between the limits of each bracket. An individual's income, including income received in kind, is used to determine the appropriate income bracket, but his contributions to the system and the financial benefits he may receive are based upon his base salary. While contributions are based upon the insured individual's ability to pay, medical services, including the most sophisticated and costly surgery, are available to insured individuals in all income classes solely on the basis of need. However, as indicated in Table 5, access to health care by dependents is limited to the wife of the insured in the case of pregnancy and to children of the insured during the first year of life.

Expansion of services—the coordinated rural health program

ICSS covers the most dynamic sectors of the economy and its services have been expanded into all departments in Colombia. The number of employees contributing to the system grew from 100,857 in 1950 to 940,443 in 1970.[40] During the same period, the number of medical consultations grew from 349, 046 to 5,189,239,[41] and the number of patients hospitalized increased from 16,404 to 185,336.[42]

With the cooperation of the Colombian Agrarian Reform Institute, (Instituto Colombiano de la Reforma Agraria—INCORA), the Ministry of Public Health, and the National University, ICSS initiated an experimental project in 1970, which was designed to extend health services to self-employed rural workers.[43] It was called the "Coordinated Rural Health Program" (Programa Coordinado de la Seguridad Social al Sector Campesino). ICSS had already extended its program to salaried workers in Quindio in 1950, a region dedicated almost exlusively to the cultivation of coffee and the coffee industry, and later to the banana zone in the north of Colombia cultivated by the United Fruit Company, and to rural workers employed in the iron works of the Paz de Rio, S.A., company in Boyacá. Under the Coordinated Rural Health Program, however, general health and maternity insurance and occupational illness and work insurance,

TABLE 6

Colombian Social Security Institute: Expenditures Under Health Insurance Programs, 1970

	EXPENDITURES		
	(in millions of pesos)	(percentage distribution)	Average per insured worker (pesos)
1. Medical and dental consultations	185.5	20.9	235.7
2. Hospitalization, surgery, obstetrics	254.9	28.7	323.9
3. Diagnosis and treatment services	40.9	4.6	52.0
4. Pharmaceutical and other supplies	87.8	9.9	111.5
5. Pecuniary benefits	55.4	6.2	70.4
6. Expenditures common to all health services	41.3	4.6	52.5
7. Expenditures on health services during previous periods	103.5	11.7	131.5
8. Administrative expenditures	63.5	7.2	80.7
9. Expenditures common to health services and administration	24.7	2.8	31.4
10. Investment expenditures	26.9	3.0	34.1
11. Service of the long term debt	3.3	0.4	4.2
TOTAL EXPENDITURES	887.8	100.0	1128.2

Source: Instituto Colombiano de Seguros Sociales, *Informe del Director General: 1.970 1.971*, p. 129.

excluding pecuniary benefits, were extended to a selected sample of self-employed rural workers and their families in the southwest region of the Department of Meta, which is situated in the eastern plains of Colombia. These workers were small landholders who had received loans from INCORA. Participation in the program was voluntary, and the costs were shared between the workers, ICSS, and INCORA. The workers paid one-third of total contributions, while ICSS and INCORA shared the other two-thirds, or the part generally paid by the employer, equally.

The programmed zone included ten municipalities with a total of about 100,000 inhabitants, 80 percent of whom lived in rural areas. The climate in this area is characterized by an average temperature of about 25 to 30 degrees centigrade and 70 to 80 percent humidity, with rain during about ten months of the year. The principal economic activities are extensive cattle ranching and agriculture, mainly the cultivation of rice, plantains, yucca, coffee, soybeans, and cotton. Gastrointestinal diseases, malnutrition, malaria, and respiratory diseases have been the most common causes of morbidity. Prior to designing and implementing the plan, a survey was carried out of the human and material medical resources available in the area as well as a complementary medical-social survey. Employees of ICSS, the Social and Preventive Medicine Department of the Medical Faculty of the National University, and supervisors and inspectors of INCORA carried out the medical-social survey. The survey was conducted, using a sample of 398 families, in order to determine the distribution of individuals by age and sex, the degree of literacy, the hygienic conditions in homes and, using a smaller sample of 25 families, to determine the most frequent causes of the need for medical care, who provides medical care, professional personnel or quacks, and the estimated cost to those who receive services.

The Ministry of Health was to cooperate in the plan directly by intensifying its preventive and eradication campaigns against prevailing endemic diseases in the region affecting both the general and the insured population, and indirectly, by making available the installations and equipment of its health institutions through its respective sectional health service. The National Hospital Fund, which is partially financed by ICSS, as mentioned earlier, was to construct, remodel, and provide equipment for health institutions in the zone.

The medical care plan elaborated comprises three levels: Rural Health Promoters, Intermediate Health Posts and Health Centers, and Hospital Centers. Rural Health Promoters were trained to work in their own communities on a virtually voluntary basis, receiving only a small monthly allowance for transportation and other expenditures. These were typically daughters of community leaders, able to read and write functionally, who were given eight week courses in health education and preventive health measures. The Rural Health Promoters would make periodic home visits, administer first aid, and facilitate the referral of patients to, or visits to patients by, the nearest health personnel.

Health Posts and Health Centers were staffed with medical and dental students in the final year of their studies and with auxiliary personnel. Medical attention at this level was to be the axis of the rural extension system; it was to moderate the current demand for curative medical services from the lowest to the highest level of health care. In addition to providing medical services, health personnel at this level were to supervise the Rural Health Promoters and the drugstores (*Boticas Comunales*), which were to sell prescribed medication at slightly more than cost, and to determine which patients needed to be remitted to Hospital Centers, which had better equipment and more qualified professional staff.

Despite promotional campaigns in all ten cities of the region, only 222 families enrolled, as compared to the 500 expected, and this resulted in underutilization of contracted facilities. The failure of more families to subscribe was attributed in part to the voluntary nature of the program, the low educational level and reserved and distrustful attitude of rural people toward collective efforts to improve social welfare, and the need to pay the entire insurance cost for the year in advance. In 1971, the program lost its experimental character, and in 1972, it was extended to the Department of Huila, where the number of participants is larger.[44]

Supporters of the program point out that it is unjust not to have a universal social security system, as the rural worker pays for the health services provided to others by ICSS through the prices of the goods that he purchases.[45] Furthermore, this program forced the rural worker to save and to make a sacrifice to obtain health services and, through the work of the Rural Promoters, he was taught to replace the "curanderos," or rural quacks, formerly consulted in case of illness, with trained medical personnel. With the cooperation of various rural institutions, such as the federations for coffee growers, cotton growers, rice planters, etc., it is hoped that the system may be extended further in the future.

Summary

The discussion in this chapter covered four areas: (1) the role of public health expenditures in the Colombian development strategy, (2) the historical evolution of health policies and institutions in Colombia, (3) the health services financed by Colombia's Ministry of Public Health in 1970, and (4) the health services provided by the Colombian Social Security Institute in 1970. Each of these is briefly summarized below.

The Colombian authorities have been following a four-pronged development strategy involving increased labor-intensive urban development; the promotion of labor-intensive export production; the encouragement of agricultural production and land redistribution; and income redistribution through progressive taxation and the expansion of social services. Health expenditures are mainly justified on the basis of their expected contribution toward reducing disparities in the distribution of income by reducing the gap in health status between upper and lower income groups.

During the 1960's the institutional structure of the health sector was improved and a National Ten-Year Health Plan covering the period 1968-1977 was drafted. A number of laws were enacted which strengthened and consolidated the control of the Ministry of Public Health over the public health system, including regional and municipal health services.

The services provided by the Ministry of Public Health in 1970 were classified as involving either health recuperation, that is, expenditures for medical-hospital care, or health promotion and protection. The most important programs pertaining to health promotion and protection were: (1) the maternal/child care program, (2) the rural and urban sanitation programs, and (3) the various vaccination campaigns and direct campaigns against tropical diseases, which were discussed under Epidemiology. While some services are provided directly by the Ministry, others are financed by the Ministry and implemented by other agencies.

The Colombian Social Security Institute provides mainly curative health care. Under its General Health and Maternity Insurance Scheme, health services are provided to employees, the wife of the insured in the case of pregnancy, and children of the insured until they become a year old. The scheme is financed by contributions by employers (two-thirds) and by employees (one-third), and to a minor extent by transfers from the Central Government and from surplus funds of the other two insurance schemes into a Solidarity Fund which is used to provide health services in economically weak regions. While social security contributions are based upon the employee's ability to pay, access to health services is based upon the patient's need. Since 1949, health services provided by ICSS have been expanded into all regions in Colombia, and in 1970, services began to be extended to self-employed rural workers.

NOTES AND REFERENCES

[1] World Bank, *Health: Sector Policy Paper* (Washington, D.C.: World Bank, 1975), pp. 25-27.

[2] USAID Mission to Colombia, "An Analysis of the Colombian Public Health Sector," Bogotá, D.E., Colombia, December 1972, pp. 157-158. (Xeroxed.)

[3] *Ibid.*, p. 159.

[4] *Ibid.*, pp. 161-162.

[5] In 1970, the Ministry of Public Health and the social security institutions, the largest of which is the Colombian Social Security Institute, accounted for an estimated 70 percent of total expenditures for public health, excluding expenditures for water and sewerage in urban areas. See *Ibid.*, p. 151; based on data included in: International Bank for Reconstruction and Development, *Economic Growth of Colombia* (Baltimore: Johns Hopkins Press, 1972), p. 429.

[6] USAID Mission to Colombia, "An Analysis of the Colombian Public Health Sector," pp. 17-18.

[7] *Ibid.*, p. 18.

[8] *Ibid.*, p. 162.

[9] Centro de Estudios sobre Desarrolo Economico (CEDE), Universidad de los Andes, *Proyecciones de la Poblacion Colombiana: 1965-85* (Bogota, D. E.: Centro de Estudios sobre Desarrollo Economico, 1968).

[10] USAID Mission to Colombia, "An Analysis," *op. cit.*, p. 19.

[11] International Bank for Reconstruction and Development, *Economic Growth of Colombia*, p. 425.

[12] USAID Mission to Colombia, "An Analysis," *op. cit.*, p. 26.

[13] A sectional health service exists for each political division of the country. It is headed by a chief of service, appointed by the Departmental Governor, and an executive board, and it is attached to the Ministry of Health through integration contracts between the Ministry and each of the sectional health services located in the departments, territories, and *intendencias* in Colombia. The functions and responsibilities of the sectional health service and its role in integrating local health services into a sector program are defined in these contracts.

[14] USAID Mission to Colombia, "An Analysis," *op. cit.*, p. 23.

[15] Ministerio de Hacienda y Credito Publico, Direccion General del Presupuesto, Division de Estudios Presupuestales, *Boletin de la*

Direccion General del Presupuesto: No 62—Diciembre de 1972 (Bogotá, D. E.: Imprenta Nacional, 1973), p. 75.

[16] USAID Mission to Colombia, "An Analysis," *op. cit.*, p. 14.

[17] *Ibid.*

[18] USAID Mission to Colombia, "An Analysis," *op. cit.*, pp. 9, 13.

[19] Rural sanitation programs are classified in part as environmental hygiene in Table 2.

[20] USAID Mission to Colombia, "An Analysis," *op. cit.*, p. 60.

[21] *Ibid.*

[22] *Ibid.*, pp. 64-65.

[23] *Ibid.*, p. 75.

[24] See *Ibid.*

[25] Instituto Nacional de Fomento Municipal, *Situacion Actual del Insfopal Dentro de las Instituciones del Sector Sanitario* (Bogotá, D. E.: Ministerio de Salud Publica, 1972), p. 2.

[26] Ministerio de Salud Publica, *informe al honorable congreso de la republica de Colombia: 1972-1973* (Bogotá, D. E.: Minsterio de Salud Publica, 1974), p. 39.

[27] Ministerio de Salud Publica and Associacion de Facultades de Medicina, *Investigacion Nacional de Morbilidad: Atención Medica* (Bogotá, D. E.: Asociacion de Facultades de Medicina and Ministerio de Salud Publica, 1968).

[28] *Ibid.*, p. 7.

[29] *Ibid.*, pp. 23-24.

[30] USAID Mission to Colombia, "An Analysis," *op. cit.*, p. 151. These account for about half of total expenditures for public health, excluding expenditures for water and sewerage in urban areas.

[31] Centro Estadistico Nacional de la Construcción, *El Poder Adquisitivo de los Salarios in Colombia: 1958-1974* (Bogotá, D. E.: Centro Estadistico Nacional de la Construcción, 1974), p. 8.

[32] Instituto Colombiano de Seguros Sociales, *Informe Estadistico: 1971* (Bogotá, D. E.: Instituto Colombiano de Seguros Sociales, 1972), p. 30.

[33] USAID Mission to Colombia, "An Analysis," *op. cit.*, p. 90.

[34] Instituto Colombiano de Seguros Sociales, *Informe Estadistico: 1971*, p. 25.

[35] Instituto Colombiano de Seguros Sociales, *Informe del Director General: 1.970-1.971* (Bogotá, D. E.: Instituto Colombiano de Seguros Sociales, 1971), p. 87.

[36] These percentages applied only to Antioquia, Valle del Cauca and Santa Marta in 1970; in Cundinamarca, Quindio and in other Local Offices, the employer contributed an amount equal to 4.0 percent of the employee's base salary and the employee contributed an amount equal to 2.0 percent of his base salary.

[37] Sources: The following laws were used: Republica de Colombia, Gobierno Nacional, *Ley 90 de 1946*, 26 December 1946, which provided for the establishment of compulsory social security and the creation of the Colombian Social Security Institute; Republica de Colombia, Ministerio del Trabajo, *Decreto Numero 2690 de 1960*, 23 November 1960, which provided the general regulations governing the General Health and Maternity Insurance scheme; Republica de Colombia, Ministerio del Trabajo, *Decreto Numero 3170 de 1964*, 21 December 1964, which provided the general regulations governing the Occupational Illness and Work Insurance scheme; Republica de Colombia, Ministerio del Trabajo, *Decreto Numero 3041 de 1966*, 19 December 1966, which provided the general regulations governing the Invalidism, Old Age, and Death Benefits insurance program.

[38] Instituto Colombiano de Seguros Sociales, *Cartilla del Seguro Social Obligatorio* (Bogotá, D. E.: Instituto Colombiano de Seguros Sociales, 1950), p. 9.

[39] Instituto Colombiano de Seguros Sociales, *Informe Financiero: 1970*, p. 381.

[40] Instituto Colombiano de Seguros Sociales, *Informe del Director General: 1.970-1.971*, p. 87.

[41] *Ibid.*, p. 106.

[42] *Ibid.*, p. 107.

[43] Horacio Parra Escobar, "Programa Coordinado de Estension de la Seguridad Social al Sector Campesino," *Seguridad Social* 20 (September-December 1971): 277-312.

[44] Horacio Parra Escobar, interview held at the Colombian Social Security Institute, Bogotá, D. E., Colombia, February 1975.

[45] *Ibid.*

Chapter 4

THE REDISTRIBUTIVE IMPACT OF PUBLIC HEALTH EXPENDITURES IN COLOMBIA ON THE DISTRIBUTION OF INCOME

Introduction

In this chapter, the benefit incidence of public health expenditures in Colombia is estimated on the basis of the conclusions which emerge from the discussion of the methodology of benefit incidence in Chapters 1 and 2; in addition, the incidence of taxes levied to finance these expenditures and the net fiscal incidence of public health expenditures in Colombia are estimated. Benefits should be evaluated on the basis of individual utility rather than the cost of providing the service. Therefore, benefit incidence is estimated on a willingness-to-pay basis, as it reflects taxpayer attitudes. Attitudes motivate people to act, as when they perceive that they are benefiting, for example, and may therefore be a more crucial measure of benefits than actual expenditure levels.[1] It is assumed that total use-of-income marginal benefits from public health services are equal to their cost, and for practical reasons, estimates of source-of-income benefits are limited to income-redistributional in-kind transfers. Benefit incidence is also estimated on a cost-of-service basis, however; this is the traditional methodology for estimating benefits and cost-of-service estimates may be regarded as more objective, since they are computed under weaker assumptions, and may, therefore, receive greater attention. As indicated in Chapter 3, the analysis is limited to health services provided by the Ministry of Public Health and the Colombian Social Security Institute, which are analyzed separately.

The Ministry of Public Health

Expenditures of the Ministry of Public Health are primarily financed by national taxes. This section of the chapter consists of four parts: (1) a description of the data used to estimate the underlying distribution of income for all households in Colombia; (2) an analysis of the incidence of national taxes in Colombia; (3) an analysis of the distribution of public health benefits by income class on both a cost-of-service basis and on a willingness-to-pay basis; and (4) an analysis of the net redistributive impact or net fiscal incidence of health services provided through the Central Government's budget. As mentioned in Chapter 1, total taxes are reduced to the level of public health expenditures and allocated among income groups according to the estimated distribution of total tax burdens.[2]

The Distribution of Income Among Colombian Households, 1970

Data on the distribution of income collected by DANE, the national statistics office, in two of its household surveys[3] were adjusted by McLure in order to estimate the underlying distribution of income in Colombia.[4] The distribution estimated by McLure is used in this study.

Income Concept

The income concept used in these surveys was described as follows:

> The income concept refers to all types of income, that is, monetary and non-monetary income received for salaried work, from independent work, as remuneration to capital and other types of income, such as retirement pensions, pecuniary assistance, income through lotteries, etc. It is useful to explain that the incomes declared by individuals have one month as a reference period and are personal incomes received before taxes.[5] (Translation mine.)

The distribution of income among urban households, 1970

The distribution of income among urban households was estimated using a survey of 3,560 households taken in late 1970. The basic data provided information on the distribution of household incomes among fourteen income classes in seven large Colombian cities. The information collected for these cities was "blown up" in such a way as to be representative of urban households in the country as a whole. Following an approach broadly suggested by Polibio Cordova,[6] McLure assumed that the income distribution pattern found in each of the seven cities was representative of the pattern found in urban areas of certain regions, generally those closest to the city concerned. The ratio of the estimated number of urban households in regions for which the city was considered to be reprsentative to the number of households in the city itself was used to expand the information collected. For each city, the absolute number of households and the income found in a given income bracket were each multiplied by this ratio. The estimated distribution of household incomes in urban areas of Colombia is presented in Table 7. This distribution indicates that whereas the bottom 45 percent of urban households receives only 15 percent of income, the top 13 percent receives about 43 percent of total urban income.

The distribution of income among rural households, 1970

For the rural sector, DANE collected data on the distribution of income among the economically active rural population. The rural distribution was adjusted to approximate a household basis using data on incomes of heads of households reported by income brackets for each educational level.[7] The calculated distribution, reported in Table 8, indicates that the bottom 45 percent of rural households receives about 13 percent of rural income while the top 13 percent receives approximately 58 percent of total rural income.[8] As McLure points out, the income distributions for urban and rural areas produce virtually identical Lorenz curves (See Figure 8.) but the estimated average absolute level of household income in urban areas (43,826 pesos per year) is over four times as large as in rural areas (10,279 pesos per year).[9]

The distribution of income among all Colombian households, 1970

The distribution of income for the nation as a whole was obtained by combining the estimated distributions for urban and rural areas. According to these results, which are reported in Table 9, the bottom 45 percent of Colombian households received roughly 14 percent of all income and the top 13 percent received about 50 percent of all income. (In 1970, average income per household was about 30,000 pesos or U.S. $1,635, assuming an exchange rate of 18.35 pesos per U.S. dollar.)

Comparing the three estimated distributions, we can see that the national income distribution is substantially less equal than either the

TABLE 7: Estimated Distribution of Income among Urban Households, 1970
(Number of households in thousands; income in billions of pesos)

Income Bracket (Pesos per year)	Number of Households	Total Income	Percentage of: Households	Percentage of: Income	Cumulative percentage of: Households	Cumulative percentage of: Income
0 - 6,000	43.3	0.20	2.1	0.2	2.1	0.2
6,000 - 12,000	257.8	2.38	12.6	2.7	14.7	2.9
12,000 - 18,000	308.9	4.56	15.1	5.1	29.9	8.0
18,000 - 24,000	309.2	6.39	15.1	7.1	45.0	15.1
24,000 - 30,000	204.9	5.44	10.0	6.1	55.0	21.2
30,000 - 36,000	153.6	5.03	7.5	5.6	62.5	26.8
36,000 - 48,000	193.1	7.91	9.5	8.8	72.0	35.6
48,000 - 60,000	148.3	7.87	7.3	8.8	79.3	44.4
60,000 - 72,000	89.7	5.87	4.4	6.6	83.6	51.0
72,000 - 84,000	74.9	5.76	3.7	6.4	87.2	57.4
84,000 - 120,000	121.0	12.10	5.9	13.5	93.1	70.9
120,000 - 180,000	75.2	10.65	3.7	11.9	96.8	82.8
180,000 - 240,000	38.1	6.51	1.9	7.3	98.7	90.1
Over 240,000	24.6	8.81	1.2	9.8	100.0	100.0
TOTAL	2042.6	89.40	100.0	100.0		

Source: Unpublished records of DANE and Charles E. McLure, Jr., "The Incidence of Colombian Taxes, 1970," Program of Development Studies, Paper No. 41 (Rice University, 1973), Table 2, p. 6.

TABLE 8: Estimated Distribution of Income among Rural Households, 1970
(Number of households in thousands; income in billions of pesos)

Income Bracket (Pesos per year)	Number of Households*	Total Income*	Percentage of: Households	Percentage of: Income	Cumulative percentage of: Households	Cumulative percentage of: Income
0 - 6,000	595.7	1.79	45.3	13.3	45.3	13.3
6,000 - 12,000	421.3	3.80	32.1	28.2	77.4	41.5
12,000 - 18,000	217.9	3.92	16.6	29.1	94.0	70.6
18,000 - 24,000	↓	↓	↓	↓	↓	↓
24,000 - 30,000	67.3	2.37	5.1	17.6	99.1	88.2
30,000 - 36,000	↓	↓	↓	↓	↓	↓
36,000 - 48,000	↓	↓	↓	↓	↓	↓
48,000 - 60,000	↓	↓	↓	↓	↓	↓
60,000 - 72,000	9.3	0.92	0.7	6.8	99.8	95.0
72,000 - 84,000	↓	↓	↓	↓	↓	↓
84,000 - 120,000	↓	↓	↓	↓	↓	↓
120,000 - 180,000	1.3	0.31	0.1	2.3	99.9	97.3
180,000 - 240,000	↓	↓	↓	↓	↓	↓
Over 240,000	1.3	0.37	0.1	2.7	100.0	100.0
TOTAL	1314.1	13.48	100.0	100.0		

*Wider income brackets for rural households than for urban households were dictated by the format of the original data. Figures are given in the top line for the several narrow brackets included in the wide ones, indicated by arrows.

Source: Polibio Cordova, *Districion de Ingresos en Colombia* (Bogota: DANE, 1971), pp. 80, 84, 88, 89, 93-95 and Charles E. McLure, Jr., "The Incidence of Colombian Taxes," Program of Development Studies, Paper No. 41 (Rice University, 1973), Table 3, estimate 3, p. 8.

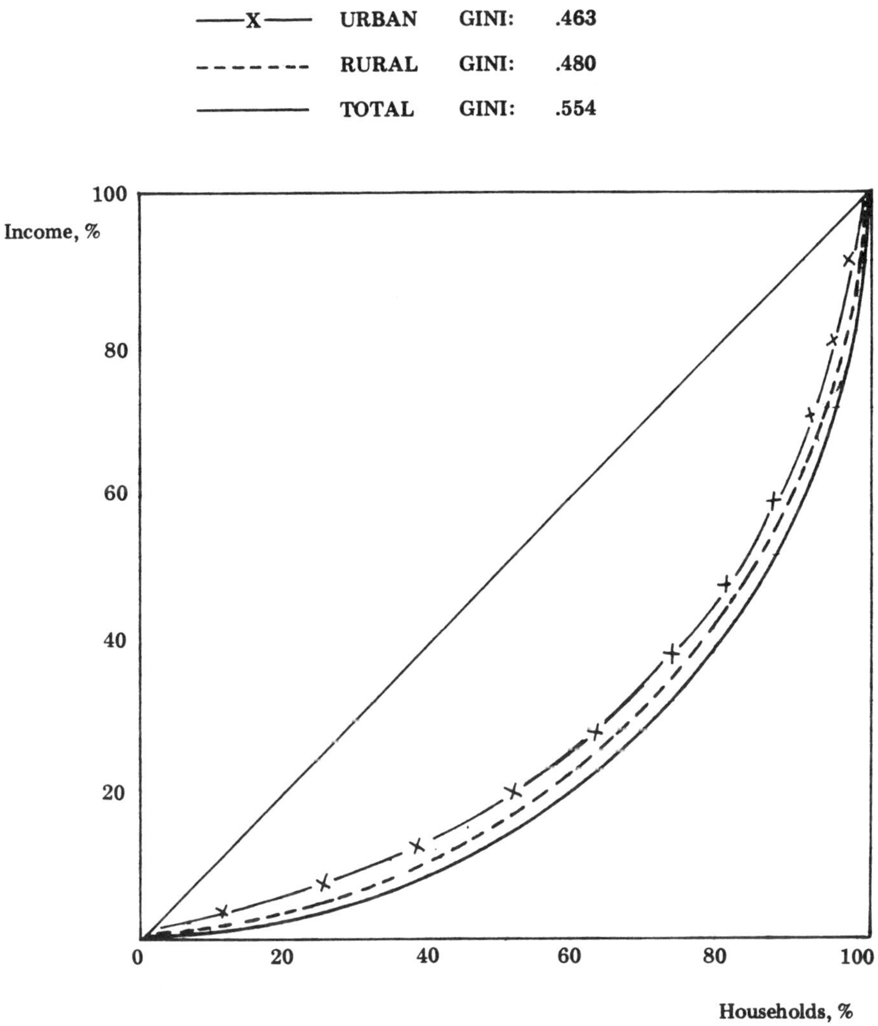

FIGURE 8: Colombia: Lorenz curves for 1970

urban or the rural distribution taken by itself. The Gini coefficient of concentration, which is the ratio of the area between the Lorenz curve and the line of equality to the triangular area under the line of equality, was estimated as 0.463 and 0.480, for the urban and rural distributions of income, respectively, and 0.554 for the distribution of income among all Colombian households in 1970.

Colombia's income distribution was compared with the distributions of income in nineteen other developed and developing countries, while recognizing that such comparisons need to be cautiously interpreted. The distribution of income in Colombia appeared to be close to the extreme in Latin America in terms of income inequality and substantially less equal than that in developed countries. In Argentina, Chile, Ecuador and Venezuela, for example, the top 10 percent of income recipients was estimated to receive about 35.8, 37.5, 30.0, and 45 percent of total income respectively, as compared to 44.0 percent in Colombia.[10]

While the survey results were accepted at face value, without questioning the extent to which the income concept used differs from economists' concept of income, several adjustments were made to them. First, assuming that corporate retained earnings enhance the economic position of shareholders and that dividends and retentions would have been higher by the amount of corporate taxes borne by shareholders, personal incomes derived from the survey data were increased by the pro-rata shares of corporate retained earnings and unshifted corporation income taxes attributable to Colombian shareholders.[11] Second, assuming that coffee export duties are borne by coffee growers and that the income of coffee growers would be higher by the amount of the tax if these duties were not imposed, the amount taken in coffee export duties and transferred to the Central Government was added to personal incomes. (McLure assumed that coffee growers probably reported income to survey interviewers net of these taxes.)[12] These adjustments are discussed further in the sections concerned with the corporate income tax and coffee export duties.

Possible errors due to the treatment of social security contributions and accrued capital gains in the income surveys need to be mentioned.[13] Both employee and employer contributions to social security should, in theory, have been included in the income reported in the surveys, according to McLure. However, the employee's share was probably only included; the data were not adjusted to correct for this possibility. Furthermore, accrued capital gains could not, as a practical matter, be included in the incomes of households, although this would have been desirable. By excluding accrued

TABLE 9: Estimated Distribution of Income Among Colombian Households, 1970
(Number of households in thousands; income in billions of pesos)

Income bracket (Pesos per year)	Number of Households	Total Income	Percentage of: Households	Income	Cumulative Percentage of: Households	Income
0-6,000	639.0	1.99	19.0	1.9	19.0	1.9
6,000-12,000	679.1	6.18	20.2	6.0	39.2	7.9
12,000-24,000	836.0	14.87	24.9	14.4	64.1	22.4
24,000-60,000	767.2	28.63	22.9	27.8	87.0	50.2
60,000-120,000	294.9	24.66	8.8	24.0	95.8	74.1
120,000-240,000	114.6	17.48	3.4	17.0	99.2	91.1
Over 240,000	25.9	9.18	0.8	8.9	100.0	100.0
TOTAL	3356.7	102.99	100.0	100.0		

Source: Tables 7 and 8.

capital gains, the extent of income inequality is probably understated and the effective tax rates for the highest income groups, for whom capital gains are likely to be significant are probably overstated.

The Distribution of National Taxes by Income Groups, 1970

To calculate the incidence of national taxes by income groups and the effective tax rates, that is, the ratio of taxes paid to total income by each income group, the major direct and indirect taxes were allocated to those income groups which are considered likely to pay them.[14] The results, in any assessment of the incidence of taxation, depend upon the availability of reliable tax data and on the hypotheses adopted concerning tax-shifting, that is, the assumptions made in regard to who, in the final analysis, bears the tax burden. The difficult problem of tax-shifting was dealt with by presenting alternative and extreme assumptions in order to provide limits within which the actual incidence of the tax system may be expected to fall.

Direct taxes

As indicated in Table 10, direct taxes consist of the personal income tax, the corporate income tax, and coffee export duties. They represented about two-thirds of total national tax collections in 1970.

Personal income tax

In allocating the personal income tax among income classes, the standard incidence assumption was made that the taxpayer upon whom the statutory liability was imposed bears the tax.[15] Unpublished tax return data for 1967, supplied by the Ministry of Finance, were used to allocate the personal income tax among income groups. The data provided referred to tax liabilities, rather than to actual tax payments, and were for the net income of individual taxpayers, rather than for the personal income of households. Therefore, several adjustments were required.

To make this series commensurable with data from the household survey, an attempt was made to aggregate the incomes of individuals in the same family who had filed separate returns, as ceding of income to one's spouse is a widespread practice in Colombia.[16] The

TABLE 10

Colombia: Total National Tax Collections by Type of Tax, 1970

	NATIONAL TAX REVENUE	
	(In millions of pesos)	(As percent of total)
Direct taxes	7563.5	65.8
Personal income tax	2927.5	25.5
Corporate income tax	3260.0	28.3
Coffee export duties[17]	1376.0	12.0
Indirect taxes[18]	3936.1	34.2
Gasoline taxes[19]	399.9	3.5
General sales tax	1089.2	9.5
Stamp taxes	539.4	4.7
Customs duties	1907.6	16.5
Total national tax revenue	11499.6	100.0

Source: McLure, "The Incidence of Colombian Taxes, 1970," pp. 17, 66.

Office of Planning of the Ministry of Finance provided a table of total amounts ceded to wives by their husbands and the number of wives who had received ceded income; the data were classified by net income classes. These data permitted estimation of the net amounts ceded to or from each income class.[20] Net amounts estimated to have been ceded by taxpayers in a given income class were added to the income figure for that class while net amounts received by taxpayers in a given income class were deducted from the income figure for that class. Then the number of wives estimated to have received ceded income in each income class was subtracted from the total number of taxpayers in each income class. In this way, the distribution of incomes recorded on tax returns was estimated by households. Taxes attributable to ceded income were then allocated to the income bracket of the husband as follows: For income groups receiving net ceded income, total tax liabilities were reduced by the estimated proportion of net ceded income to total income of the income class; then this amount was allocated to those income groups which had reported net ceding of income in proportion to the net amounts estimated as having been ceded. The adjustment for ceding made relatively little difference, except for the lowest income group, for which net income and total tax liability were significantly lower after the adjustment; as expected, those in lower income groups were net recipients of income ceded by those in higher income groups.[21]

Although income ceded to wives and subject to the highest income tax rates probably came more than proportionately from husbands in the highest income brackets, no attempt was made to correct for this defect of the procedure. Furthermore, the procedure adopted is only satisfactory for wives whose only income is that ceded by their husbands; if the wife has other income, the adjustments made reduce the number of taxpayers in her income class by one and the income in her income class by the amount ceded to her, but the wife's non-ceded income is not subtracted from the income in that income class. Since a relatively small amount of income was involved, an analysis of this problem was not undertaken. Finally, in the case of wives filing tax returns without any ceded income and other family members filing tax returns, it was not possible to consolidate these returns into family units.

The unpublished tax return data supplied for 1967 were also adjusted for growth and inflation.[22] The basic data included the number of taxpayers, net income, and total tax liability by net income brackets, as mentioned above. In order to allow for inflation and growth in average productivity, the limits of the net income brackets were multiplied by the ratio of national income per capita in 1970 to that in 1967; this was estimated at 1.49. Then the adjusted 1967 figures for tax liabilities in each income bracket were increased by a uniform fraction in order to make the total coincide with figures in the national income accounts for direct taxes levied on households in 1970 and the adjusted amount was allocated to urban households by income class, making the standard incidence assumption that these are only, or mainly, collected in urban areas. The results indicated that the personal income tax contributes importantly to the progressivity of the tax system, with effective tax rates ranging from zero for the lowest income group to about 12, 13, or 16 percent for the highest income group, depending upon the assumption adopted regarding the incidence of the corporation income tax.[23]

The corporation income tax

The incidence of the corporation income tax was analyzed under three extreme assumptions: (A) that it is borne by upper income Colombian shareholders, that is, those with incomes of 120,000 pesos per year and over; (B) that it is shifted to Colombian consumers; and (C) that it is borne by non-Colombian shareholders.[24] As mentioned earlier, personal incomes derived from the survey data were adjusted to reflect retained earnings and unshifted corporation income taxes attributable to Colombian shareholders. In case (A), it was assumed that, in the absence of the tax, an amount equal to the tax would have been available to upper income households; retained earnings were also allocated to Colombian shareholders, using the same assumption. In case (B), that is, if the tax is shifted to consumers, the survey data understate the economic income of Colombian households only by the amount of retained earnings attributable to Colombian shareholders. Finally, the income data reported in the surveys would not have to be increased if Colombian corporations were entirely owned by foreigners, as assumed in case (C). To summerize, under assumption (A) the income reported in the surveys was adjusted for both retained earnings and the corporation income tax; under assumption (B) income was adjusted only for retained earnings; and under assumption (C) the distribution of income is as reported in Table 9.[25]

In allocating the corporation income tax to income classes, the assumptions adopted were as follows. Under alternative (A), the more progressive assumption concerning the incidence of the tax, it was assumed that the tax is borne by Colombian shareholders in the top two income brackets; the results indicated effective tax rates of about 7.8 percent and 12.7 percent for the two highest income groups, in ascending order.[26] Under alternative (B), it was assumed that the tax is shifted to consumers roughly in proportion to their non-food expenditures, and the results indicated that it is borne approximately in proportion to income at an effective tax rate of about 3 percent for all income groups.[27]

Coffee export duties

In 1970, taxes levied upon coffee exports amounted to 2,821.2 million pesos, of which 1,376 million pesos flowed into central government revenue.[28] The latter figure does not include the one fifth of the coffee export tax and the other two principal taxes on the coffee sector, the retention tax and the pasilla, which are paid directly to the National Coffee Fund to finance the activities of the coffee sector.[29] Whereas taxes flowing back into the coffee sector could reasonably be ignored, those which go into general revenue should be treated as any other tax, but they should also be treated as a potential addition to household income. The income of coffee growers would be higher by approximately the amount of the tax, if these duties were not imposed. Therefore, as mentioned earlier, the amount taken in coffee export duties and transferred to the central government needs to be included at each income level of the rural income distribution. Using data on the number of coffee plantings and the value of production, by size of plantings, estimates were made of the value of coffee production and export duties by income classes.[30]

The allocation of export duties among income brackets indicated that these constitute a progressive tax element within the rural sector. For the nation as a whole, however, they are regressive. The results indicated that coffee export duties take 3.2 percent of rural income at the bottom of the income scale but 38 and 36.2 percent of rural income at the two highest income levels, in ascending order.[31]

Indirect taxes

Indirect taxes, as indicated in Table 10, consist of gasoline taxes, the general sales tax, stamp taxes, and customs duties. In 1970, they represented about one-third of total national tax revenue. The consumption patterns reported in the DANE household budget survey were used to allocate national indirect taxes separately among income groups.

Gasoline taxes

Estimated use of motor fuel was used to allocate gasoline taxes among income classes.[32] (Gasoline taxes were estimated net of the petroleum subsidy implicit in the differential exchange rate for petroleum.)[33] It was assumed that half of these taxes should be attributed to private automobile users; they were allocated among income brackets in urban and rural areas on the basis of estimated household expenditures on gasoline by income class according to the household budget survey for the seven cities; these figures were blown up using the same methodology used for the income figures, in order to estimate a national total. It was assumed that 15 percent of these taxes should be attributed to municipal buses, and these were allocated among urban households on the basis of data in the budget survey for purchases of transport services by income class. Another 15 percent was attributed to intermunicipal buses and allocated to rural households by income class under the assumption that rural households in each income bracket spent the same proportion of income on intermunicipal bus transportation as urban households do, according to the consumption survey. Finally, 20 percent of these taxes was attributed to cargo carriers and allocated across income classes on the basis of estimated expenditures on total consumption for the seven cities, which were blown up to a national total in the same way that gasoline consumption figures were. Effective gasoline tax rates were found to be slightly progressive.

Customs duties and stamp taxes

As detail on the breakdown of customs duties by commodity classes was unfortunately not available, these were allocated on the basis of non-food consumption expenditures and the same allocative guide was used for national stamp taxes. Effective tax rates for customs duties and stamp taxes were found to be slightly regressive.[34]

The national sales tax

The national sales tax consisted of a 3 percent standard rate and differential rates of 8, 10, and 15 percent. Non-food consumption expenditures were used as a basis for allocating collections produced by the standard rate. The 10 percent rate, which applied only to domestically produced cigarettes, was allocated following a procedure analogous to that for private gasoline use. The 8 and 15 percent rates applied to a number of luxury items, including automobiles, watches, electric hand appliances, imported clothes, liquors, and cigarettes, etc. Data on automobile purchases by income class was used to allocate revenues from these two rates in order to reflect the general luxury nature of the items taxed and also to compensate for having neglected the unknown luxury content of import duties. Whereas effective sales tax rates were found to be slightly regressive at low income levels, reflecting the allocation in proportion to non-food consumption expenditures in the estimation procedure, they were found to be progressive at the upper end of the income scale, reflecting the allocation of collections at the two highest rates in proportion to purchases of automobiles by income class.[35]

Total tax revenue

The analysis of direct taxes and indirect taxes needs to be combined in order to examine the incidence of taxation by the national government on all Colombian households. Table 11 reports the absolute amounts of taxes estimated to have been borne by each income group in the nation as a whole. Effective tax rates are reported separately in Table 12 for each of the assumptions regarding the incidence of the corporation income tax.

Table 12 indicates that the Colombian tax system was found to be progressive, the degree of progressivity ranging from mild to fairly strong, depending upon the assumption adopted concerning the incidence of the corporation income tax. The overall system appears to be mildly progressive, if the corporate tax is borne by foreigners (Alternative C), with the progressivity primarily attributable to the progressivity of the personal income tax, although the luxury elements of the sales tax and of customs duties also contribute to it. Progressivity appears to be considerably stronger if the corporation income tax is borne by Colombian shareholders (Alternative A) rather than by Colombian consumers (Alternative B) or by foreigners (Alternative C).

The Distribution of Benefits Generated by Health Expenditures of the Ministry of Public Health by Income Class, 1970

To estimate the incidence of the benefits generated by health expenditures of the Ministry of Public Health in 1970, the major expenditure categories were allocated to income groups using the cost-of-service methodology and the willingness-to-pay methodology. The allocative assumptions adopted for the various expenditures

TABLE 11: Allocation of National Taxes Among Households
(millions of pesos)

		Income Bracket (thousands of pesos per year)							
		0-6	6-12	12-24	24-60	60-120	120-140	Over 240	Total
Personal Income Tax		22.4	11.7	52.5	360.8	473.1	515.9	1491.1	2927.5
Corporation Income Tax:	A	-	-	-	-	-	1640.0	1620.0	3260.0
	B	89.3	167.3	458.0	918.3	720.2	577.9	317.7	3248.5
	C	-	-	-	-	-	-	-	-
Coffee Export Duties		59.0	112.0	191.0	352.0	255.0	191.0	216.0	1376.0
Indirect Taxes									
Gasoline Tax		13.7	53.7	24.4	70.5	107.3	92.9	37.4	399.9
General Sales Tax		25.0	45.9	129.0	240.7	205.9	238.9	203.7	1089.2
Stamp Taxes		14.8	27.8	76.0	152.5	119.6	96.0	52.7	539.4
Customs Duties		52.5	98.2	268.9	539.2	422.9	339.3	186.5	1907.6
Total Indirect Taxes		105.9	225.6	498.4	1002.9	855.6	767.1	480.4	3936.2
TOTAL	A	187.3	349.3	741.9	1715.7	1583.7	3114.0	3807.5	11499.7
	B	276.6	516.6	1199.9	2634.0	2303.9	2051.9	2505.2	10328.2
	C	187.3	349.3	741.9	1715.7	1583.7	1474.0	2187.5	8239.7

Source: McLure, "The Incidence of Colombian Taxes. 1970." p. 66, with the exception of export duties, which were adjusted to consist of only those duties received by the Central Govenment.

TABLE 12: Effective Rates of National Taxation, All Households

Income Bracket (pesos per year)	Alternative A[1]			Alternative B[2]			Alternative C[3]		
	Income[4] (billions of pesos)	Allocation of Taxes (millions of pesos)	Effective Rates of Taxation	Income[5] (biliions of pesos)	Allocation of Taxes (millions of pesos)	Effective Rates of Taxation	Income[6] (billions of pesos)	Allocation of Taxes (millions of pesos)	Effective Rates of Taxation
0-6,000	2.05	187.3	9.1	2.05	276.6	13.5	2.05	187.3	9.1
6,000-12,000	6.29	349.3	5.6	6.29	516.6	8.2	6.29	349.3	5.6
12,000-24,000	15.06	741.9	4.9	15.06	1199.9	8.0	15.06	741.9	4.9
24,000-60,000	28.99	1715.7	5.9	28.99	2634.0	9.1	28.99	1715.7	5.9
60,000-120,000	24.92	1583.7	6.4	24.92	2303.9	9.2	24.92	1583.7	6.4
120,000-240,000	21.01	3114.0	14.8	19.37	2051.9	10.2	17.67	1474.0	8.3
Over 240,000	12.72	3807.5	29.9	11.10	2505.2	22.6	9.39	2187.5	23.3
TOTAL	111.04	11499.7	10.4	107.78	11488.1	9.6	104.37	8239.7	7.9

[1]Corporation income tax is borne by Colombian shareholders
[2]Corporation income tax is shifted to consumers
[3]Corporation income tax is borne by foreigners
[4]Income is adjusted for export duties, retained earnings, and the corporate income tax
[5]Income is adjusted for export duties and retained earnings
[6]Income is adjusted for coffee export duties

Source: McLure, "The Incidence of Colombian Taxes, 1970." p. 18; and Table 11.

are indicated below. As indicated in Chapters 1 and 2,[36] the capital stock in the health sector generates a flow of services over time; however, no attempt was made to impute an annual value to services from public hospitals and other capital facilities of the health sector already in place or from new capital facilities. Current and investment expenditures were combined in making both sets of estimates and it was assumed, as in the Snodgrass study cited in Chapter 2, that these estimates may be interpreted as indicative of future changes in the distribution of consumption benefits from health services.

Cost-of-Service estimates

The benefits from health services estimated on a cost-of-service basis and allocated by income class are displayed in Table 13. As in previous benefit incidence studies in which the cost-of-service methodology was employed, costs were allocated to those "on whose behalf" it was assumed that they had been incurred.

Allocative assumptions

Expenditures on maternal-child care programs and other social services were allocated to the two lowest income groups, as data concerning the socio-economic characteristics of women who requested family planning services in 1970 indicated that the monthly family income of these beneficiaries was 825 pesos, on average.[37] Expenditures on sanitary services and epidemiology were treated as pure public goods; a malarial swamp or a polluted water supply both constitute central sources of infection, the elimination of which provides benefits indiscriminately to all inhabitants of the given area. Therefore, expenditures on sanitary services provided in rural and urban areas were allocated in proportion to the estimated distribution of households by income class in rural and urban areas, respectively, and expenditures on the epidemiology of communicable diseases were allocated in proportion to the estimated distribution of total households by income class. Medical-hospital expenditures were allocated on the basis of information on private health care patterns of expenditures contained in the 1970 survey of household expenditure patterns in the seven cities.[38] The survey results give some indication of public as well as private health services received, as most public health services generally require the recipient to pay at least some small charge for services provided. (The principal results of this survey in regard to the level and pattern of expend-

TABLE 13: Ministry of Public Health: Distribution of Health Service Benefits by Income Class — Cost-of-Service Basis

Income Brackets (Pesos per year)	Medical-Hospital Care	Maternal-Child Care	Epidemiology	Sanitary Services		Administrative and Technical Services	Total Benefits			
				Rural	Urban		(millions of pesos)	% of total	% of income	pesos per household
	(in millions of pesos)									
0-6,000	7.9	159.3	33.1	38.1	6.3	34.6	279.3	21.4	14.0	437.1
6,000-12,000	38.6	169.1	35.2	27.0	38.0	42.0	349.9	26.9	5.7	515.2
12,000-24,000	76.8	-	43.3	16.2	91.3	20.7	248.3	19.0	1.7	297.0
24,000-60,000	158.1	-	39.9	2.5	103.3	34.2	338.0	25.9	1.2	440.6
60,000-120,000	-	-	15.3	0.2	42.2	2.6	60.3	4.6	0.2	204.5
120,000-240,000	-	-	5.9	1.1	16.5	1.0	23.5	1.8	0.1	205.1
Over 240,000	-	-	1.4	0.1	3.6	0.2	5.3	0.4	-	204.6
TOTAL	281.4	328.4	174.1	84.2	301.2	135.3	1304.6	100.0	1.3	

itures on health services are discussed in Appendix 2.) Expenditures on medical-hospital care were allocated in proportion to the distribution of households by income class which received medical consultations in 1970 and whose annual incomes were 60,000 pesos or less.[39] It was assumed that those with incomes exceeding 60,000 pesos had received private medical care.[40] Finally, expenditures on administrative and technical services were allocated in proportion to the distribution of benefits from programs classified under Public Health in Table 2 in Chapter 3.

Distribution of benefits

The incidence of health service benefits was found to be sharply regressive, that is, pro-poor, over all income classes, with benefits as a percent of income falling from 14.0 percent for the lowest income class to about one-tenth of one percent and less than that for the two highest income classes in ascending order. Absolute benefits per household were estimated to be about 477 pesos, on average, for the two lowest income classes, which account for 40 percent of total households, but only about 205 pesos, on average, for the three highest income groups.

Willingness-to-Pay estimates

The benefits from health services estimated on a willingness-to-pay basis and imputed by income class are presented in Table 14. To recapitulate some of the main points discussed in Chapters 1 and 2, in order to measure the benefits generated by health services, Mishan argued that the individual's willingness-to-pay for a reduction in the risk of contracting disease should be used to measure his welfare gain due to the provision of health programs. Aaron and McGuire showed that in order to impute the benefits from public services by income class, value in exchange estimates must be established. To do this, citizen attitudes toward particular public health services must be known; individual evaluations must be based upon empirical data. In order to utilize the theorem developed by Aaron and McGuire, Maital proposed a general functional form for the marginal utility of income and estimated particular values of the crucial parameter, namely the income elasticity of marginal utility, for various countries. Greene, Neenan, and Scott employed the general functional form proposed by Maital and a value of the income elasticity of marginal utility equal to one in order to impute use-of-income benefits by income class. They inferred this value of

TABLE 14: Ministry of Public Health: Distribution of Health Service Benefits by Income Class — Willingness-to-Pay Basis

Income Bracket (pesos per year)	Medical-Hospital Care	Maternal-Child Care			Epidemiology	Sanitary Services		Administrative and Technical Services	Total Benefits			
		Source-of-Income	Use-of-Income	Total		Rural	Urban		(millions of pesos)	(% of Total)	(% of Income)	pesos per household
	(In millions of pesos)											
0-6,000	10.7	159.3	-	159.3	3.3	11.1	0.6	21.1	206.2	12.6	10.4	322.7
6,000-12,000	33.8	169.1	-	169.1	10.5	23.7	8.1	26.0	271.2	16.6	4.4	399.4
12,000-24,000	81.0	-	51.6	51.6	25.2	26.3	38.0	19.2	241.3	14.8	1.6	288.6
24,000-60,000	155.9	-	99.4	99.4	48.4	17.3	89.2	37.1	447.3	27.4	1.6	583.0
60,00-120,000	-	-	85.1	85.1	41.6	2.6	81.6	15.4	226.3	13.9	0.9	767.4
120,000-240,000	-	-	60.1	60.1	29.4	2.2	55.7	10.8	158.2	9.7	0.9	1380.5
Over 240,000	-	-	32.2	32.2	15.7	0.9	28.0	5.8	82.6	5.0	0.9	3189.2
TOTAL	281.4	328.4	328.4	656.8	174.1	84.2	301.2	135.4	1633.1	100.0		

the income elasticity of marginal utility, or the willingness-to-pay index, from Fellner's analysis complemented by survey and voting data; the income elasticity of marginal utility was also assumed to have a value of one in this study. (To test the sensitivity of the results to the value of the income elasticity of marginal utility chosen, alternative values of the index [1.5 and 2.0] were also used.) This method, as indicated in Chapter 1, was used not only to impute use-of-income, public benefits across income classes, but also to impute use-of-income, private benefits to those income classes which were assumed to benefit from particular services.[41] Since a precise quantitative evaluation of particular services is not feasible, the estimates of benefits based upon the evidence that is available may only be regarded as accurate within a range of values.

The procedures that were used to estimate benefits from public health expenditures and to impute them by income class may be summarized as follows: (1) source-of-income benefits from in-kind transfers were imputed to recipients on a cost basis; (2) use-of-income benefits from health expenditures were classified as either public redistributive benefits, public nonredistributive benefits, or private benefits and the monetary value of use-of-income benefits was assumed to equal total expenditures; (3) public nonredistributive benefits was allocated to all households on a cost basis and then imputed by income class using the assumption that the income elasticity of marginal utility is one; (4) private benefits were first allocated to the recipients of market-like benefits from certain health services, such as curative health care; then these benefits were imputed across those income classes again assuming that the elasticity of marginal utility with respect to income is one; (5) public redistributive benefits were assigned to income classes that were assumed to have been willing and able to finance redistributive services for others, that is, they were allocated to those who were assumed to have an effective demand for providing in-kind transfers to others; they were then allocated across those income classes under the assumption that the elasticity of marginal utility with respect to income is one. The specific assumptions that were made regarding each of the health expenditure categories will now be discussed.

Allocative assumptions

Since maternal-child care programs and other social services are designed to provide in-kind transfers to low income individuals, it must be concluded that the recipients of these transfers should be exempt from any tax liability to finance these programs. Therefore, recipients of in-kind transfers were imputed source-of-income benefits from these redistributive programs on the basis of their cost. As indicated earlier, the average monthly household income of beneficiaries in 1970 was about 825 pesos, or 9,900 pesos annually; source-of-income benefits were, therefore, imputed to the two lowest income classes. Furthermore, assuming an optimal provision of these programs, use-of-income public redistributive benefits equal to the monetary value of the source-of-income benefits were imputed to households with income above 12,000 pesos annually, that is, to those households that were assumed to have an effective demand for providing these programs.

Expenditures on sanitary services in rural and urban areas and expenditures on epidemiology were assumed to generate use-of-income public nonredistributive benefits. The former were imputed indiscriminately to all inhabitants of rural and urban areas, respectively, while the latter were imputed indiscriminately to all citizens, that is, across all income classes.

Expenditures on medical-hospital care were allocated to those income groups that received medical consultations in 1970, namely the first four income classes from the bottom, as determined in making the cost-of-service estimates.

The remaining expenditures on administrative and technical services were allocated across income classes in proportion to the distribution of total benefits from programs listed under Public Health in Table 3, Chapter 3.[42]

Distribution of benefits

The incidence of health benefits measured on a willingness-to-pay basis was found to be regressive, that is, pro-poor, over all income classes, as in the cost-of-service estimates.[43] Benefits as a percent of income declined from 10.4 percent for the lowest income group, as compared to 14.0 percent when benefits were measured on a cost-of-service basis, to 0.9 percent for the highest income group, as compared to less than 0.1 percent in the case of cost-of-service estimates. Absolute benefits per household were also correspondingly lower for the two lowest income groups when benefits were measured on a willingness-to-pay basis, 361 pesos per household as compared to 477 pesos per household on a cost-of-service basis, while they were strikingly different for the three highest income groups, 1,779 pesos per household as compared to 205 pesos per household on a cost-of-service basis. While the cost-of-service estimates, made on the assumption that the marginal utility of income is constant across income classes, represent the extreme case of the most pro-poor benefit incidence pattern, the willingness-to-pay estimates indicate a significantly less pro-poor incidence pattern. This is attributable to two assumptions: first, that the marginal utility of income declines proportionately with income, and second, that maternal-child care programs generate public redistributive benefits for upper income groups.

The Net Fiscal Incidence of Health Expenditures of the Ministry of Public Health by Income Class, 1970

Fiscal residuals describe the overall incidence of fiscal activities by the government on income groups.[44] They measure the excess of benefits generated by public services over taxes paid for each income class.

Table 15 presents fiscal residuals which were calculated on the basis of cost-of-service estimates of benefits and estimates of taxes paid by income class, using only assumptions A and B, or the most and the least progressive assumptions concerning the incidence of the corporation income tax in order to bracket the true tax incidence. Net fiscal residuals and net fiscal residuals per household were found to be largest for the two lowest income classes and negative for those with incomes in excess of 60,000 pesos per year. Furthermore, the incidence of fiscal residuals was found to be regressive, that is, residuals as a percentage of money income decline monotonically over all income classes, with the highest income class having the most negative percentage.

The welfare gain or loss that an income class receives due to the tax and expenditure activities of the government, evaluated at the margin, is what the pattern of fiscal residuals derived from the willingness-to-pay estimates of benefits purports to represent. The pattern of fiscal residuals which emerged using benefits estimated on a willingness-to-pay basis and the distribution of taxes paid according to assumptions A and B is presented in Table 16.[45] In this case, the incidence was also found to be regressive. However, net fiscal residuals and net fiscal residuals per household were found to be less favorable to lower income classes and more favorable or less unfavorable to middle and upper income classes.

The Colombian Social Security Institute

The Colombian Social Security Institute (Instituto Colombiano de Seguros Sociales—ICSS) finances health services for affiliated

TABLE 15: Ministry of Public Health: Net Fiscal Residuals by Income Class — Benefits Estimated on a Cost-of-Service Basis

Income Brackets (pesos per year)	Total Benefits Received	Total Taxes Paid (A)	Total Taxes Paid (B)	Net Fiscal Residual (A)	Net Fiscal Residual (B)	Net Fiscal Residual per Household (A)	Net Fiscal Residual per Household (B)	Net Fiscal Residual as a percent of income (A)	Net Fiscal Residual as a percent of income (B)
	(In millions of pesos)					(In pesos)			
0-6,000	279.3	20.9	31.3	258.4	248.0	+404.4	+388.1	13.0	12.5
6,000-12,000	349.9	39.1	58.7	310.8	291.2	+457.7	+428.8	5.0	4.7
12,000-24,000	248.3	84.8	135.7	163.5	112.6	+195.6	+134.7	1.1	0.8
24,000-60,000	338.0	194.4	298.8	143.6	39.2	+187.2	+ 51.1	0.5	0.1
60,000-120,000	60.3	180.0	262.2	-119.7	-201.9	-405.9	-684.6	- 0.5	-0.8
120,000-240,000	23.5	353.5	233.5	-330.0	-210.0	-2879.0	-1832.5	-1.9	-1.2
Over 240,000	5.3	431.8	284.4	-426.5	-279.1	-16467.2	-10776.1	-4.6	-3.0
TOTAL	1304.6	1304.6	1304.6						

TABLE 16: Ministry of Public Health: Net Fiscal Residuals by Income Class — Benefits Estimated on a Willingness-to-Pay Basis

Income Brackets (pesos per year)	Total Benefits Received	Total Taxes Paid (A)	Total Taxes Paid (B)	Net Fiscal Residual (A)	Net Fiscal Residual (B)	Net Fiscal Residual per Household (A)	Net Fiscal Residual per Household (B)	Net Fiscal Residual as a percent of income (A)	Net Fiscal Residual as a percent of income (B)
	(In millions of pesos)					(In pesos)			
0-6,000	206.2	20.9	31.3	185.3	174.9	+290.0	+273.7	9.3	8.8
6,000-12,000	271.2	39.1	58.7	232.1	212.5	+341.8	+312.9	3.8	3.4
12,000-24,000	241.3	84.8	135.7	156.5	105.6	+187.2	+126.3	1.1	0.7
24,000-60,000	447.3	194.4	298.8	252.9	148.5	+329.6	+193.6	0.9	0.5
60,000-120,000	226.3	180.0	262.2	46.3	-35.9	+157.0	-121.7	0.2	-0.1
120,000-240,000	158.2	353.5	233.5	-195.3	-75.3	-1704.2	-657.1	-1.1	-0.4
Over 240,000	82.6	431.8	284.4	-349.2	-201.8	-1348.3	-7791.5	-3.8	-2.2
TOTAL	1633.1	1304.6	1304.6						

employees and eligible dependents primarily with contributions to the General Health and Maternity Insurance Program (El Seguro Social Obligatorio de Enfermedad No Profesional y Maternidad) by employers and employees. The employer and the employee pay two-thirds and one-third, respectively, of the contributions to this program. As mentioned in Chapter 3, General Health and Maternity Insurance has been compulsory for all private sector employees since 1949, whereas the Occupational Illness and Work Insurance and the Invalidism, Old Age and Death Benefits programs were introduced in 1965 and 1967, respectively. In 1970, 86 percent of the revenues channeled through this program originated in contributions, while 11 percent were derived from central government transfers to the Solidarity Fund, and 3 percent constituted small transfers mainly from the disability program and to a minor extent from the retirement program. Table 17 indicates the distribution of revenue available to provide medical care in 1970 by source. The remaining sections of this chapter include: (1) a discussion of the distribution of income among employees insured by ICSS; (2) an analysis of the distribution of social security contributions to finance health services by income class; and (3) an analysis of the distribution of benefits generated by expenditures on health services by income class both on a cost-of-service basis and on a willingness-to-pay basis; and (4) an analysis of the net fiscal incidence of health services provided through the Colombian Social Security Institute.

The Distribution of Income Among Colombian Workers Insured by ICSS, 1970

Tables 18 and 19 indicate the estimated distribution of mainly private sector employees insured by ICSS in 1970 by income class and by both income class and the economic activity in which they were employed, respectively. For the purpose of making social security contributions, as mentioned in Chapter 3, income is defined to include wage and salary earnings as well as income received in kind.

The distribution of income among employees insured by ICSS appears to be very different from the national distribution of income. The data in Table 18 indicate that whereas the bottom 45 percent of employees received about 20 percent of all income, the top 13 percent received about 38 percent; furthermore, the Gini coefficient of concentration was estimated as 0.403. According to the national income distribution, the bottom 45 percent only received about 14 percent of all income and the top 13 percent received

TABLE 17: Colombian Social Security Institute: Revenues for General Health and Maternity Services, 1970 (in millions of pesos)

Regional and Local Offices	Antioquia, Valle del Cauca, Santa Marta	Cundinamarca, Quindio, Local Offices	TOTAL
A. Contributions	349.2	384.1	733.3
1. Employer	232.8	256.0	488.8
2. Employee	116.4	128.1	244.5
B. Solidarity Fund	7.8	86.0	93.8
C. Transfers from Disability Program	10.1	16.5	26.6
TOTAL	367.1	486.6	853.7

Source: Instituto Colombiano De Seguros Sociales, *Informe Del Director General: 1.970-1.971* (Bogota, D.E.: Instituto Colombiano de Seguros Sociales, 1971), p. 177.

50 percent, as mentioned earlier. This difference may be attributed to the limited coverage by ICSS of workers employed in agriculture. The data indicate that the primary sector only provided 9 percent of insured workers, whereas the secondary and the tertiary sectors provided 48 percent and 44 percent, respectively. They also indicate that the largest proportion of insured workers was employed in manufacturing industries (41 percent) and the second largest proportion was employed in commerce (22 percent). Finally, the distribution of workers by both income class and economic activity indicates that in the primary and tertiary sectors, most workers are located in the second and third income brackets from the bottom, whereas in the secondary sector, the largest number of workers is concentrated in the third and fourth income brackets from the bottom.

The Distribution of Social Security Contributions by Income Class, 1970

Social security contributions are, in fact, not contributions but rather involuntary payroll taxes without exemptions or deductions. Various views have been offered regarding the incidence, particularly of the employer contribution, of this tax. For example, Milton Friedman regards the employer contribution as a tax that is paid in the long run by the employee out of his wages.[46] On the other hand, others, such as George Jaszi[47] and Harold M. Groves[48] have held an agnostic view regarding the incidence of the employer tax. Groves has written that:

> The incidence of these taxes cannot be predicted with any great degree of assurance. On the whole the safe conclusion would seem to be that it is divided among employers, labor and consumer; but in what proportion cannot definitely be said.[49]

John A. Brittain attempted to assess the long-run incidence of the employer share of social security taxes.[50] In his theoretical analysis, he dealt with the supply of labor, while in his empirical analysis, he was concerned with quantitatively isolating the impact of the employers' tax on real wage rates in the long run. His conclusion from the theoretical and the empirical analysis is that social security payroll taxes are entirely borne by labor. The theoretical case for this conclusion is based upon acceptance of the concept of a demand curve for labor and the notion that the employer is indifferent to what the sums that he must pay in order to hire labor are called. To hire N units of labor of a given quality, the employer is willing

TABLE 18: ESTIMATED DISTRIBUTION OF INCOME AMONG WORKERS INSURED BY ICSS, 1970
(Number of Workers and Income in Thousands)

Income Bracket (pesos per month)	No. of Workers	Total Monthly Income	Percentage of: Workers	Percentage of: Income	Cumulative Percentage of: Workers	Cumulative Percentage of: Income
0-359.99	37.5	11237	4.0	0.96	4.0	0.96
360.00-539.99	181.7	81772	19.3	6.96	23.3	7.92
540.00-779.99	206.8	136460	22.0	11.62	45.3	19.54
780.00-1,079.99	154.5	143716	16.4	12.24	61.7	31.78
1,080.00-1,499.99	129.0	166409	13.7	14.17	75.4	45.95
1,500.00-2,039.99	105.0	185814	11.2	15.82	86.6	61.77
2,040.00-2,819.99	51.3	124749	5.5	10.62	92.1	72.39
2,820.00-3,779.99	29.4	96970	3.1	8.26	95.2	80.65
3,780.00-5,039.99	19.8	87534	2.1	7.46	97.3	88.11
5,040.00 and over	25.4	139616	2.7	11.89	100.0	100.00
TOTAL	940.4	1174277	100.0	100.0		

TABLE 19: Colombian Social Security Institute: Number of Insured Workers By Economic Activity and Income Bracket, 1970

Economic Activity \ Income Bracket	0-359.9	360-539.9	540-779.9	780-1,079.9	1,080-1,499.9	1,500-2,039	2,040-2,819	2,820-3,779.9	3,780-5,039.9	5,040 & over	Total
Primary sector	5046	29789	21642	10741	7883	3873	1138	406	259	307	81444
Agriculture, hunting and fishing											
Extractive industries											
Secondary Sector	8627	68205	107925	80734	71473	57755	27129	11754	6838	9133	449393
Manufacturing industries											(381557)
construction											(49862)
Electricity, gas, water and sanitary services											(14974)
Tertiary sector	23423	83902	77190	63058	49643	43352	23070	17225	12752	15991	409606
Commerce											202963
Transportation, communicating, storage											46288
Services											140567
Other											19788
TOTAL	37456	181716	206757	154533	128999	104980	51337	29385	19849	25431	940443

Source: Same as for Table 17, pp. 94, 96.

to pay a certain price, as indicated by the demand curve, and whether, in part, the price is labeled the employer's contribution does not make any difference; if he were required to pay both the employer's as well as the employee's contribution, he would reduce the nominal wage, that is, the total compensation less the employer tax, accordingly. Brittain argues that the employer could not be expected to pay more total real compensation for a given amount of labor if he were suddenly required to pay both components of the tax, except in the case of some short run qualifications, such as a labor contract. If, in addition, the aggregate labor supply curve is assumed to be totally inelastic, he concludes that both components of the social security payroll taxes are borne by labor and aggregate employment, or the cost of labor, are unaffected. In other words, the total pretax compensation to labor will be reduced by the two components of the tax at the fixed employment level. He argues that the tax would also not produce an employment effect if the supply of labor were elastic, if labor bargained on the basis of total compensation, including both components of the tax, rather than in terms of net income after taxes. However, if two conditions prevailed, namely that both the supply price failed to include the employer's contribution and the supply of labor were not totally inelastic, he argues that there would be an employment effect due to the employer's attempt to recover the tax by lowering the basic wage. The effect on real compensation to labor would depend upon both the elasticity of demand and the elasticity of the supply of labor functions.[51] He does not consider this case a significant qualification of his general proposition. He rejects the former condition, supporting the position that it doesn't matter to the worker whether he receives a higher net wage or the employer pays a higher tax contribution. He argues that "this result depends on labor's viewing one withheld tax as part of its income but not the other."[52] He finds "this behaviour . . . difficult to rationalize."[53] Implicitly, Brittain is considering income taxes and the employees' share of the tax as net income and both as borne by labor and is concluding that therefore the employers' share must also be borne by labor.[54]

Using cross section regression models based on the CES function (constant elasticity of substitution production function) and cross-section data on value-added, wages and salaries, and employment, and effective payroll tax rates estimated on the basis of statutory rates, Brittain also attempted to isolate quantitatively the impact of the employers' tax on real wage rates in the long run. The main conclusion was that ". . . given the level of productivity in a country, the presence of a payroll tax on employers tends to reduce the wage in dollars by roughly the amount of the tax."[55]

In his response to Brittain's study, Feldstein criticizes both the theoretical and the empirical analysis.[56] He argues that even if it were true that the tax does not affect the quantity of labor supplied, it would not be true, as Brittain concludes, that labor bears the burden of the tax, because the capital stock and relative prices are affected by the tax. In examining the basis for the conclusion that the quantity of labor supplied would not be affected, Feldstein poses what he regards as the relevant question, namely what the effect of the tax would be if the supply of labor were elastic. In Brittain's analysis, he concludes that even if the labor supply were elastic, the quantity of labor supplied would be unaffected by the tax, if labor bargained in terms of total compensation. Feldstein points out that this implies the implausible assumption that at each gross wage, the quantity of labor supplied would not change as a result of a change in the share of the gross wage allocated for taxes. He also indicates that this was due to an error in Brittain's analysis. Brittain concentrated on the employer's share of the tax and assumed that employees regard their share of the tax as equal to part of their income and therefore that this share is borne by employees. This led him to the conclusion that there was no reason to treat the two components of the tax differently and that the employers' tax must also be paid by labor. He finds unacceptable Brittain's assumption that the employee does not treat his share of the tax as a reduction from his income. Feldstein also criticizes Brittain's failure to consider the effect of the social security program on capital accumulation and in his comments upon the empirical analysis, he concludes that the regressions provide no basis for the conclusion that was reached.[57] He states that "his conclusion that the entire burden of the tax is borne by labor is not supported by either the theoretical discussion or the regression analysis. At most, his empirical analysis has shown that, *if* the supply of labor and capital were not changed by the tax, the working of the factor markets would cause the entire burden to fall on labor."[58]

In his reply, Brittain states that ". . . I judge Feldstein to be less than 100 percent in error."[59] However, he makes a number of points, including the following: (1) the second sentence of the statement by Feldstein that was quoted above is exactly what he claims to have shown in the empirical analysis; (2) the aggregate labor supply only needs to be approximately inelastic or the supply price of labor only needs to approximately include the full amount of the tax for most of the tax to be borne by labor; (3) real wages could be depressed, as Feldstein points out, by the capital formation effect of the social security programs, and (4) he states that "in sum, my empirical finding that the payroll tax comes out of the real demand price of labor has considerable significance if one accepts my a priori suggestions that employment effects are probably minor."[60]

Theoretically, agreement has not been reached on whether the tax generally (1) reduces wages, (2) reduces profits, or (3) raises prices. In the empirical analysis shown in Table 22, the methodology adopted by Gillespie was followed.[61] In a developing country, such as Colombia, it appears likely, due to the weak labor market, that the worker bears his share of the tax; it also appears likely that half of the employer's share of the tax would be shifted backward to the laborer, while the other half might be shifted forward to the consumers of luxury goods, who are generally in the upper income groups.

As mentioned in Chapter 3, contributions to the General Health and Maternity Insurance Program are paid according to a scale of absolute weekly amounts by income level and constituting a uniform percentage of income.[62] In 1970, one scale of rates applied to the sectional offices of Cundinamarca and Quindio and local offices, with the exception of Santa Marta, while another, higher scale of contributions, applied to the sectional offices of Antioquia, Valle del Cauca, and the local office of Santa Marta. These scales are shown separately in Tables 20 and 21, respectively. Data were available for the total number of man-years in 1970 (every 52 weeks of contributions represented a worker) corresponding to each sectional and local office of ICSS, and these were separated into the two groups for which the scales for making contributions were applicable.[63] Then, using information available for 1971 concerning the distribution of workers by income class and by sectional and local offices,[64] these were distributed separately across income classes. The appropriate scale of rates was then used to allocate the employee's and half of the employer's share to the various income classes. As total employee contributions estimated in this manner exceeded total actual contributions by 12 percent, the actual total was allocated among income classes using the estimated distribution of contributions. The other half of total employer contributions was allocated to ICSS employees by income class on the basis of the distribution of consumption expenditures by income class, according to the seven-cities survey by DANE (with interpolations to fit brackets in ICSS data), although the burden of these is probably also partially borne by workers not insured by ICSS as well. The small proportion of revenues transferred from the disability program, which is financed through employer contributions, also was allocated on the basis of total consumption expenditures by income groups.

Contributions to the Solidarity Fund, which consist in part of

INSTITUTO COLOMBIANO DE SEGUROS SOCIALES
TABLE 20
CATEGORIAS DE SALARIOS Y APORTES
VIGENTES DESDE EL 10 DE SEPTIEMBRE DE 1965 — DECRETO NO 1825 DE 1965

TABLA DE CATEGORIAS

Categoria	Salario Diario		Salario Semanal		Salario Mensual	
	De	Hasta	De	Hasta	De	Hasta
I	$ —	$ 11.99	$ —	$ 83.99	$ —	$ 359.9
II	12.00	17.99	84.00	125.99	360.00	539.9
III	18.00	25.99	126.00	181.99	540.00	779.9
IV	26.00	35.99	182.00	251.99	780.00	1.079.9
V	36.00	49.99	252.00	349.99	1.080.00	1.499.9
VI	50.00	67.99	350.00	475.99	1.500.00	2.039.9
VII	68.00	93.99	476.00	657.99	2.040.00	2.819.9
VIII	94.00	125.99	658.00	881.99	2.820.00	3.779.9
IX	126.00	167.99	882.00	1.175.99	3.780.00	5.039.9
X	168.00	y más	1.176.00	y más	5.040.00	y má

SEGURO DE ENFERMEDAD NO PROFESSIONAL Y MATERNIDAD
APORTES DISCRIMINADOS POR SEMANAS
(Cajas Seccionales de Antioquia y Valle del Cauca y Oficina Local de Santa Marta)

Cat.	No. de Semanas Cotizadas	Aportes			Cat.	No. de Semanas Cotizadas	Aportes		
		Patrono	Trabajador	Total			Patrono	Trabajador	Tot
	1	3.30	1.65	4.95		1	18.80	9.40	28.2
	2	6.60	3.30	9.90		2	37.60	18.80	56.4
I	3	9.90	4.95	14.85	VI	3	56.40	28.20	84.6
	4	13.20	6.60	19.80		4	75.20	37.60	112.8
	5	16.50	8.25	24.75		5	94.00	47.00	141.0
	1	5.00	2.50	7.50		1	26.10	13.05	39.1
	2	10.00	5.00	15.00		2	52.20	26.10	78.3
II	3	15.00	7.50	22.50	VII	3	78.30	39.15	117.4
	4	20.00	10.00	30.00		4	104.40	52.20	156.6
	5	25.00	12.50	37.50		5	130.50	65.25	195.7
	1	7.30	3.65	10.95		1	35.40	17.70	53.1
	2	14.60	7.30	21.90		2	70.80	35.40	106.2
III	3	21.90	10.95	32.85	VIII	3	106.20	53.10	159.3
	4	29.20	14.60	43.80		4	141.60	70.80	212.4
	5	36.50	18.25	54.75		5	177.00	88.50	265.5
	1	10.30	5.15	15.45		1	48.76	24.38	73.1
	2	20.60	10.30	30.90		2	97.52	48.76	146.2
IV	3	30.90	15.45	46.35	IX	3	146.28	73.14	219.4
	4	41.20	20.60	61.80		4	195.04	97.52	292.5
	5	51.50	25.75	77.25		5	243.80	121.90	365.7
	1	14.10	7.05	21.15		1	61.50	30.75	92.2
	2	28.20	14.10	42.30		2	123.00	61.50	184.5
V	3	42.30	21.15	63.45	X	3	184.50	92.25	276.7
	4	56.40	28.20	84.60		4	246.00	123.00	369.0
	5	70.50	35.25	105.75		5	307.50	153.75	461.2

MINISTERIO DEL TRABAJO Y SEGURIDAD SOCIAL
INSTITUTO COLOMBIANO DE SEGUROS SOCIALES
TABLE 21
CATEGORIAS DE SALARIOS Y APORTES
VIGENTES DESDE EL 10 DE SEPTIEMBRE DE 1965 — DECRETO NO 1825 DE 1965

TABLA DE CATEGORIAS

Categoria	Salario Diario		Salario Semanal		Salario Mensual	
	De	Hasta	De	Hasta	De	Hasta
I	$ —	$ 11.99	$ —	$ 83.99	$ —	$ 359.99
II	12.00	17.99	84.00	125.99	360.00	539.99
III	18.00	25.99	126.00	181.99	540.00	779.99
IV	26.00	35.99	182.00	251.99	780.00	1.079.99
V	36.00	49.99	252.00	349.99	1.080.00	1.499.99
VI	50.00	67.99	350.00	475.99	1.500.00	2.039.99
VII	68.00	93.99	476.00	657.99	2.040.00	2.819.99
VIII	94.00	125.99	658.00	881.99	2.820.00	3.779.99
IX	126.00	167.99	882.00	1.175.99	3.780.00	5.039.99
X	168.00	y más	1.176.00	y más	5.040.00	y más

SEGURO DE ENFERMEDAD NO PROFESIONAL Y MATERNIDAD
APORTES DISCRIMINADOS POR SEMANAS PARA LAS
Cajas Seccionales de Cundinamarca y Quindio y Oficinas Locales (Excepto Santa Marta)

Cat.	No. de Semanas Cotizadas	Aportes			Cat.	No. de Semanas Cotizadas	Aportes		
		Patrono	Trabajador	Total			Patrono	Trabajador	Total
	1	2.80	1.40	4.20		1	16.52	8.26	24.78
	2	5.60	2.80	8.40		2	33.04	16.52	49.56
I	3	8.40	4.20	12.60	VI	3	49.56	24.78	74.34
	4	11.20	5.60	16.80		4	66.08	33.04	99.12
	5	14.00	7.00	21.00		5	82.60	41.30	123.90
	1	4.20	2.10	6.30		1	22.68	11.34	34.02
	2	8.40	4.20	12.60		2	45.36	22.68	68.04
II	3	12.60	6.30	18.90	VII	3	68.04	34.02	102.06
	4	16.80	8.40	25.20		4	90.72	45.36	136.08
	5	21.00	10.50	31.50		5	113.40	56.70	170.10
	1	6.16	3.08	9.24		1	30.80	15.40	46.20
	2	12.32	6.16	18.48		2	61.60	30.80	92.40
III	3	18.48	9.24	27.72	VIII	3	92.40	46.20	138.60
	4	24.64	12.32	36.96		4	123.20	61.60	184.80
	5	30.80	15.40	46.20		5	154.00	77.00	231.00
	1	8.68	4.34	13.02		1	41.16	20.58	61.74
	2	17.36	8.68	26.04		2	82.32	41.16	123.48
IV	3	26.04	13.02	39.06	IX	3	123.48	61.74	185.22
	4	34.72	17.36	52.08		4	164.64	82.32	246.96
	5	43.40	21.70	65.10		5	205.80	102.90	308.70
	1	12.04	6.02	18.06		1	51.24	25.62	76.86
	2	24.08	12.04	36.12		2	102.48	51.24	153.72
V	3	36.12	18.05	54.18	X	3	153.72	76.86	230.58
	4	48.16	24.08	72.24		4	204.96	102.48	307.44
	5	60.20	30.10	90.30		5	256.20	128.10	384.30

Ver Al Rispaldo

some of the tax revenue collected by the central government, should be allocated in part to the private sector employees affiliated with ICSS and in part also to other taxpayers. This breakdown is not available but these revenues constitute a small proportion of the total. They were allocated across income classes according to the distribution of total national taxes under assumption B, with interpolations to fit brackets. Medical care centers in zones with little economic activity and with few, low paid workers, generate high service and administrative costs in relation to the number of people to be protected; the inadequate revenues of these economically weak regions, as mentioned in Chapter 3, are bolstered by transfers from the Solidarity Fund.[65]

Tables 22 and 23 indicate the allocation by income class of social security contributions and other taxes levied in order to finance health services provided by ICSS and the estimated effective rates of taxation by income class, respectively. Effective rates of social security and other taxes combined, as shown in Table 23, were found to be slightly progressive over most income ranges and strongly progressive at the top of the scale. The observed progressivity is largely attributable to the incidence of employer contributions allocated on the basis of total consumption expenditures in urban areas and to a lesser extent to the incidence of national taxes transferred to the Solidarity Fund. Effective tax rates including only employee contributions and employer contributions assumed to have been borne by employees illustrate the approximate proportionality with respect to income intended by decrees governing social security contributions.

The Distribution of Benefits Generated by Health Expenditures of the Colombian Social Security Institute by Income Class, 1970

Socio-economic information on the beneficiaries of health services provided by ICSS is scarce and difficult to acquire. To obtain this information, ICSS used reports on income subsidies paid to insured workers in 1971. These income payments partially compensate workers for wages lost due to absence from work on account of illness or work-related accidents. Physicians employed by ICSS must approve the payment of these subsidies, which are calculated as indicated in Table 5 of Chapter 3.[66] These reports were used to retrieve income data on individual beneficiaries from ICSS' files and to compile information concerning the nature and duration of the illness, and the age, sex, and occupation of the patient. For obvious reasons physicians were reluctant to request income information

TABLE 22: Colombian Social Security Institute: Allocation of Social Security Contributions and Other Sources of Revenue Among Affiliated Workers By Income Class, 1970

I. CUDINAMARCA, QUINDIO, AND LOCAL OFFICES

Income Bracket (Pesos per year)	Number of Man-Years	Employee Contributions Total (In millions of pesos)	Employee Contributions (% of total)	Employee Contributions Adjusted Total	Employer Contributions (Absorbed by wages) (in millions of pesos)	Employer Contributions (Shifted to Consumers)	Employer Contributions Total	Solitary Fund	Transfers from Disability Program	Grand Total
0-4,319.99	18561	1.35	0.9	1.15	1.15	3.20	4.35	0.86	0.41	6.77
4,320-6,479.99	73791	8.06	5.5	7.04	7.04	2.05	9.09	1.72	0.26	18.11
6,480-9,359.99	104121	16.68	11.4	14.59	14.59	3.46	18.05	1.72	0.44	34.80
9,360-12,959.99	75601	17.06	11.7	14.98	14.98	4.35	19.33	2.58	0.56	37.45
12,960-17,999.99	58399	18.28	12.5	16.00	16.00	6.02	22.02	4.30	0.77	43.09
18,000-24,479.99	51155	21.97	15.1	19.33	19.33	4.74	24.07	5.16	0.61	49.17
24,480-33,839.99	27615	16.28	11.2	14.34	14.34	8.45	22.79	6.02	1.09	44.24
33,840-45,359.99	16297	13.05	8.9	11.39	11.39	11.78	23.17	6.88	1.52	42.96
45,360-60,479.99	11318	12.11	8.3	10.62	10.62	7.68	18.30	9.46	0.99	39.37
60,480 and over	15845	21.11	14.5	18.56	18.56	76.29	94.85	47.31	9.82	170.54
TOTAL	452703	145.96	100.0	128.00	128.00	128.00	256.00	86.02	16.48	486.50

II. ANTIOQUIA, VALLE DEL CAUCA, SANTA MARTA

Income Bracket (Pesos per year)	Number of Man-Years	Employee Contributions Total (In millions of pesos)	Employee Contributions (% of total)	Employee Contributions Adjusted Total	Employer Contributions (Absorbed by wages) (in millions of pesos)	Employer Contributions (Shifted to Consumers)	Employer Contributions Total	Solitary Fund	Transfers from Disability Program	Grand Total
0-4,319.99	5101	0.44	0.3	0.35	0.35	2.91	3.26	0.08	0.25	3.94
4,320-6,479.99	55766	7.25	5.6	6.52	6.52	1.86	8.38	0.16	0.16	15.22
6,480-9,359.99	75828	14.39	11.2	13.04	13.04	3.14	16.18	0.16	0.27	29.65
9,360-12,959.99	54065	14.48	11.3	13.15	13.15	3.96	17.11	0.23	0.34	30.83
12,960-17,999.99	51005	18.70	14.5	16.88	16.88	5.47	22.35	0.39	0.47	40.09
18,000-24,479.99	46925	22.94	17.8	20.72	20.72	4.31	25.03	0.47	0.37	46.59
24,480-33,839.99	23802	16.15	12.5	14.55	14.55	7.68	22.23	0.54	0.67	37.99
33,840-45,359.99	10881	10.01	7.8	9.08	9.08	10.71	19.79	0.62	0.93	30.42
45,360-60,479.99	6801	9.62	6.7	7.80	7.80	6.98	14.78	0.85	0.60	24.03
60,480 and over	9860	15.77	12.3	14.32	14.32	69.37	83.69	4.27	6.01	108.29
TOTAL	34004	128.75	100.0	116.40	116.40	116.40	232.80	7.76	10.08	367.05

TABLE 23: Colombian Social Security Institute: Effective Rates of Social Security Taxation and Other Taxes Levied in Order to Finance Health Services Through the Colombian Social Security Institute, 1970

Income Bracket	Income		Social Security Contributions and Other Sources of Financing				Effective Rates of Taxation	
(pesos per year)	Unadjusted	Adjusted[1]	I[2]	II[3]	Total	(% of Total)	(1)[4]	(2)[5]
	(millions of pesos)							
0-4,319.99	134.8	136.3	6.77	3.94	10.71	1.3	7.9	2.2
4,320-6,479.99	981.3	994.9	18.11	15.22	33.33	3.9	3.4	2.8
6,480-9,359.99	1637.5	1665.1	34.80	29.65	64.45	7.6	3.9	3.4
9,360-12,959.99	1724.6	1752.7	37.45	30.83	68.28	8.0	3.9	3.3
12,960-17,999.99	1996.9	2029.8	43.09	40.09	83.18	9.8	4.1	3.3
18,000-24,479.99	2229.8	2269.9	49.17	46.59	95.76	11.2	4.2	3.6
24,480-33,839.99	1497.0	1525.0	44.24	37.99	82.23	9.6	5.4	5.9
33,840-45,359.99	1163.6	1184.1	42.96	30.42	73.38	8.6	6.2	3.5
45,360-60,479.99	1050.4	1068.8	39.37	24.03	63.40	7.4	5.9	3.5
60, 480 and over	1675.4	1708.3	170.54	108.29	278.83	32.7	16.3	3.9
TOTAL	14091.3	14335.7	486.50	367.05	853.55	100.0	6.0	3.5

[1] Adjusted for the unshifted portion of social security contributions by employers.
[2] Cundinamara, Quindio, and Local Offices. (See table 22).
[3] Antioquia, Valle del Cauca, Santa Marta. (See table 22).
[4] Total sources of financing: social security contributions, Solidarity Fund, and transfers from the disability program.
[5] Employee contributions and employer contributions assumed to have been borne by employees.

Sources: Tables 18 and 22.

directly from their patients. Consequently, available data refer only to cases and days of incapacity, rather than to cases of illness. To estimate the incidence of the benefits generated by health expenditures of ICSS in 1970, as mentioned earlier, total expenditures were allocated to income groups using both the cost-of-service methodology and the willingness-to-pay methodology.

Cost-of-Service estimates

Table 24 presents the distribution of benefits from health services by income class estimated on a cost-of-service basis. Costs were allocated across income classes in proportion to the distribution of total days of incapacity by income class, as shown in Table 25. This was necessary because the expenditure categories indicated in Table 6, Chapter 3,[67] do not coincide with the various causes of illness classified by income class in Table 26. (ICSS uses a system of disease classification by the system of the body affected, whereas in the discussion of expenditures by the Ministry of Public health, the emphasis was upon the epidemiological view of communicable diseases, or how diseases are transmitted. The latter approach facilitates understanding of the relationship between poverty and disease.) Therefore, expenditures for hospitalization and surgery, for example, and for other categories listed in Table 6 could not be allocated separately by income class.

The results indicate that the incidence of health service benefits is sharply regressive. Benefits decline as a percent of income from 23.1 percent for the lowest income group to 0.6 percent for the highest income group. However, estimated benefits per worker were highest for the third, fourth, and fifth income groups from the bottom. These three income groups account for 58 percent of total benefits.

The statistics compiled by ICSS contain a great deal of useful information concerning the recipients of health services provided by ICSS, and this information could be used to design programs to reduce the incidence of illness by income group, occupation, sex, age, and also in intermediate and small cities, for which the data are also available. (See Tables 25 to 30.) Authors of previous benefit incidence studies have rarely had such a wealth of information available to them concerning the characteristics of beneficiaries. McLure,[68] De Wulf,[69] and others have been stressing the need for more detailed empirical work on the characteristics of beneficiaries than has thus far been done in previous benefit incidence studies, so that better programs may be designed to assist those strata of the population who need these services most.

TABLE 24: Colombian Social Security Institute: Distribution of Health Service Benefits By Income Class, 1970

Income Bracket (pesos per year)	Health Service Benefits: Cost of Service Basis				Health Service Benefits: Willingness-to-Pay Basis			
	(millions of pesos)	% of total	% of income	pesos per worker	(millions of pesos)	% of total	% of income	pesos per worker
0-4,319.99	31.1	3.5	23.1	829	8.5	1.0	6.3	227
4,320-6,479.99	155.4	17.5	15.8	855	62.1	7.0	6.3	342
6,480-9,359.99	212.2	23.9	13.0	1026	103.0	11.6	6.3	498
9,360-12,959.99	166.9	18.8	9.7	1080	108.3	12.2	6.3	701
12,960-17,999.99	137.6	15.5	6.9	1067	126.1	14.2	6.3	978
18,000-24,479.99	99.4	11.2	4.5	947	140.2	15.8	6.3	1335
24,480-33,839.99	45.3	5.1	3.0	883	94.1	10.6	6.3	1834
33,340-45,359.99	19.5	2.2	1.7	663	73.7	8.3	6.3	2507
45,360-60,479.99	10.7	1.2	1.0	540	66.6	7.5	6.3	3364
60,480 and over	9.8	1.1	0.6	386	104.8	11.8	6.3	4164
TOTAL	887.8	100.0	6.3	944	887.8	100.0	6.3	944

The data appear to reveal some correlation between a worker's social position, as measured by his income, and his tendency to become ill. Some of the information provided in Tables 25 to 30 concerning recipients of health services provided by ICSS, and the poorest recipients, in particular, may be summarized as follows:

(1) Whereas the distribution of days of incapacity and the distribution of cases of incapacity are roughly similar to the distribution of workers by income bracket, the average number of days per case declines continuously as income rises over the five lowest income brackets, remains constant over the following two brackets, and then begins to rise again. (See Table 25.)

(2) The most frequent causes of days of incapacity among all income groups are shown in Tables 26 and 27 to be poisoning and violence (37 percent), which includes fractures, burns, adverse effects due to chemicals and other wounds; complications related to pregnancy, childbirth, and post-delivery period (17 percent); and diseases of the digestive apparatus (6 percent). Among lower income groups, days of incapacity are largely attributable to complications related to pregnancy, childbirth and the post-delivery period. Whereas this group of causes accounts for about 26 percent of days of incapacity among the two lowest income groups, its relative importance declines continuously as income increases so that for the highest income group it only represents about 5 percent of days of incapacity. The second and third most important causes of incapacity for the two lowest income groups are poisoning and violence (25 percent) and diseases of the digestive apparatus (6 percent), respectively; the latter includes ulcers, appendicitis, intestinal obstructions and hernia, illnesses related to the dental structure, and other diseases of the digestive apparatus. The relative importance of diseases of the digestive apparatus declines continuously as income increases over the first five income classes from the bottom and then increases in relative importance for upper income groups, accounting for over 11 percent of days of incapacity for the two highest income groups.

(3) About 45 percent of the cases of incapacity are among workers between the ages of 20 and 39, with an average duration of about 14 days per case, while only about 16 percent of cases of incapacity are attributable to those over the age of 40, but the average number of days per case is about 17. (See Table 28; as shown in the table, in a significant proportion of cases, the patient's age was not specified.)

(4) Manufacturing industries account for the greatest percentage of both cases and days of incapacity among the economic sectors in which workers insured by ICSS are employed. As shown in Tables 29 and 30, manufacturing industries, which include 41 percent of

TABLE 25: Colombian Social Security Institute: Number of Days and Cases of Incapacity by Income Class, 1970

Income Bracket (pesos per month)	DAYS		CASES		Average Number of Days per Case
	Number	Percent of total	Number	Percent of total	
0-359.99	94908	3.5	4119	2.4	23.0
360.00-539.99	479751	17.5	25418	14.6	18.9
540.00-779.99	655017	23.9	40793	23.5	16.1
780.00-1,079.99	514840	18.8	34390	19.8	15.0
1,080.00-1,499.99	425715	15.5	30469	17.5	14.0
1,500.00-2,039.99	306975	11.2	21223	12.2	14.5
2,040.00-2,819.99	139473	5.1	9795	5.6	14.2
2,820.00-3,779.99	61845	2.2	4025	2.3	15.4
3,780.00-5,039.99	32402	1.2	1890	1.1	17.1
5,040.00 and over	32230	1.1	1735	1.0	18.6
TOTAL	2743156	100.0	173857	100.0	15.8

Source: Instituto Colombiano de Segura Sociales, *Estadistica de Casos de Incapacidad Con Subsidios Pagados: Suplemento al Informe Estadistico: Año de 1971* (Bogotá, D.E.: Instituto Colombiano de Seguros Sociales, 1972), pp. 18-19.

Groups of Causes	I Up to 359 Cases	Days	II 360 to 539 Cases	Days	III 540 to 779 Cases	Days	IV 780 to 1,079 Cases	Days	V 1,080 to 1,499 Cases	Days
I. Infections and Parasitic Diseases	232	5015	1439	23832	1818	27046	1466	19470	1233	15552
II. Tumors (Neoplasmas)	77	2004	329	8654	382	8481	291	5829	269	5111
III. Gland, Endocr. Nutric. and Metabolic Diseases	28	525	129	2791	153	3294	91	2058	111	2259
IV. Diseases of the Blood and Blood Producing Organs	13	190	83	1164	75	1211	36	813	27	357
V. Mental Disorders	69	2298	400	10246	566	16860	448	11847	398	9698
VI. Diseases of the Nervous System and Sensory Organs	207	2967	1014	16616	1484	22743	1201	16914	1160	15311
VII. Diseases of the Circulatory Apparatus	205	5049	851	21251	885	20509	678	17827	590	13247
VIII. Diseases of Respiratory Apparatus	406	4317	1990	17384	2602	19311	2411	17916	2252	15719
IX. Diseases of the Digestive Apparatus	330	7574	1636	29462	2136	36467	1668	26703	1398	22243
X. Diseases of the Genitourinary Apparatus	249	3993	1167	17313	1334	17806	1082	13821	989	13093
XI. Comp. Related to Pregnancy, Childbirth and the Post-Delivery Period	746	32741	3011	119078	3006	119613	1956	79357	1426	60828
XII. Diseases of the Skin and the Celular Tissue under the Skin	202	1989	1374	12105	1958	15328	1536	12317	1306	10302
XIII. Diseases of the Osteomuscular System and the Connecting Tissue	194	4388	1167	22247	1622	25465	1438	23599	1412	21997
XIV. Congenital Anomalies	2	35	32	684	30	708	34	691	27	558
XV. Certain Peri. Causes of Morbidity and Mortality	-	-	-	-	-	-	-	-	-	-
XVI. Badly Defined Symptoms and Diseased States	306	5240	3043	49827	3506	50445	3523	50428	3625	47893
XVII. Poisoning and Violence	853	16583	7753	127097	19236	269730	16531	215250	14246	171547
TOTAL	4119	94908	25418	479751	40793	655017	34390	514840	30469	425915

Groups of Causes	VI 1,500 to 2,039 Cases	Days	VII 2,040 to 2,819 Cases	Days	VIII 2,820 to 3,779 Cases	Days	IX 3,780 to 5,039 Cases	Days	X 5,040 and over Cases	Days
I. Infections and Parasitic Diseases	815	9052	347	3431	187	2093	91	1277	112	1619
II. Tumors (Neoplasmas)	190	3914	100	2205	42	625	25	589	34	753
III. Gland. Endocr. Nutric, and Metabolic Diseases	67	1542	51	750	17	281	27	527	16	596
IV. Diseases of the Blood and Blood Producing Organs	20	391	-	-	1	20	3	28	-	-
V. Mental Disorders	325	8292	154	3206	61	1510	38	821	48	1169
VI. Diseases of the Nervous System and Sensory Organs	778	10876	358	5675	187	3227	104	1778	98	1822
VII. Diseases of the Circulatory Apparatus	443	9622	217	4235	118	2149	79	2183	86	2340
VIII. Diseases of the Respiratory Apparatus	1583	12255	782	5664	342	2325	183	1266	177	1506
IX. Diseases of the Digestive Apparatus	1038	17386	493	8285	253	4614	185	3807	204	3647
X. Diseases of the Genitourinary Apparatus	663	8650	347	3750	152	1745	87	1239	75	1240
XI. Comp. Related to Pregnancy, Childbirth and the Post-Delivery Period	662	37363	343	14663	128	6067	64	2802	36	1566
XII. Diseases of the Skin and the Celular Tissue Under the Skin	771	6623	363	2964	142	1003	69	809	55	527
XIII. Diseases of the Osteomuscular System and the Connecting Tissue	976	14980	571	9122	272	4725	139	2155	125	2289
XIV. Congenital Anomalies	12	158	8	173	5	89	-	-	1	12
XV. Certain Peri. Causes of Morbidity and Mortality	-	-	-	-	-	-	-	-	-	-
XVI. Badly Defined Symptoms and Diseased States	3208	44862	1406	18646	578	8874	286	4361	287	4692
XVII. Poisoning and Violence	9472	121009	4255	56704	1540	22498	510	8760	381	8452
TOTAL	21223	306975	9795	139473	4025	61845	1890	32402	1735	32230

Source: Instituto Colombiano de Seguros Sociales, *Estadistica de Casos de Incapacidad Con Subsidios Pagados: Supplemento Informe Estadistico: Año de 1971* (Bogotá, D.E.: Instituto Colombiano de Seguros Sociales, 1972), pp. 28-29.

TABLE 27: Colombian Social Security Institute: Number of Cases and Days of Incapacity By Groups of Causes and Income Bracket, 1970 (percentage distribution)

Groups of Causes	I Up to 359 Cases	I Up to 359 Days	II 360 to 539 Cases	II 360 to 539 Days	III 540 to 779 Cases	III 540 to 779 Days	IV 780 to 1,079 Cases	IV 780 to 1,079 Days	V 1,080 to 1,499 Cases	V 1,080 to 1,499 Days
I. Infections and Parasitic Diseases	5.6	5.3	5.7	5.0	4.5	4.1	4.3	3.8	4.0	3.7
II. Tumors (Neoplasmas)	1.9	2.1	1.3	1.8	0.9	1.3	0.8	1.1	0.9	1.2
III. Gland Endocr. Nutrit and Metabolic Diseases	0.7	0.6	0.5	0.6	0.4	0.5	0.3	0.4	0.4	0.5
IV. Diseases of the Blood & Blood Producing Organs	0.3	0.2	0.3	0.2	0.2	0.2	0.1	0.2	0.1	0.1
V. Mental Disorders	1.7	2.4	1.6	2.1	1.4	2.6	1.3	2.3	1.3	2.3
VI. Diseases of the Nervous System and Sensory Organs	5.0	3.1	4.0	3.5	3.6	3.5	3.5	3.3	3.8	3.6
VII. Diseases of the Circulatory Apparatus	5.0	5.3	3.3	4.4	2.2	3.1	2.0	3.5	1.9	3.1
VIII. Diseases of the Respiratory Apparatus	9.9	4.5	7.8	3.6	6.4	2.9	7.0	3.5	7.4	3.7
IX. Diseases of the Digestive Apparatus	8.0	8.0	6.4	6.1	5.2	5.6	4.9	5.2	4.6	5.2
X. Diseases of the Genitourinary Apparatus	6.0	4.2	4.6	3.6	3.3	2.7	3.1	2.7	3.2	3.1
XI. Comp. Related to Pregnancy, Childbirth and the Post-Delivery Period	18.1	34.5	11.8	24.8	7.4	18.3	5.7	15.4	4.7	14.3
XII. Diseases of the Skin and the Cellular Tissue under the Skin	4.9	2.1	5.4	2.5	4.8	2.3	4.5	2.4	4.3	2.4
XIII. Diseases of the Osteomuscular System and the Connecting Tissue	4.7	4.6	4.6	4.6	4.0	3.9	4.2	4.6	4.6	5.2
XIV. Congenital Anomalies	-	-	0.1	0.1	0.6	0.1	0.1	0.1	0.1	0.1
XV. Certain Peri. Causes of Morbidity and Mortality	-	-	-	-	-	-	-	-	-	-
XVI. Badly Defined Symptoms and Diseased States	7.4	5.5	12.0	10.4	8.6	7.7	10.2	9.8	11.9	11.3
XVII. Poisoning and Violence	20.7	17.5	30.5	26.5	47.2	41.2	48.1	41.8	46.8	40.3
TOTAL	100.0	100.0	100.0	100.0	100.0	100.0	100.0	100.0	100.0	100.0

TABLE 27 (continued): Colombian Social Security Institute:
Number of Cases and Days of Incapacity By Groups of Causes and Income Bracket, 1970
(percentage distribution)

Groups of Causes	VI 1,500 to 2,039		VII 2,040 to 2,819		VIII 2,820 to 3,779		IX 3,780 to 5,039		X 5,040 & over		All Income Brackets	
	Cases	Days	Cases	Days	Cases	Days	Cases	Days	Cases	Days	Cases	Days
I. Infections and Parasitic Diseases	3.8	2.9	3.5	2.5	4.6	3.4	4.8	3.9	6.5	5.0	4.5	4.0
II. Tumors (Neoplasmas)	0.9	1.3	1.0	1.6	1.0	1.0	1.3	1.8	2.0	2.3	1.0	1.4
III. Gland Endocr. Nutrit and Metabolic Diseases	0.3	0.5	0.5	0.5	0.4	0.5	1.4	1.6	0.9	1.8	0.4	0.5
IV. Diseases of the Blood & Blood Producing Organs	0.1	0.1	-	-	-	-	0.2	0.1	-	-	0.1	0.2
V. Mental Disorders	1.5	2.7	1.6	2.3	1.5	2.4	2.0	2.5	2.8	3.6	1.4	2.4
VI. Diseases of the Nervous System and Sensory Organs	3.7	3.5	3.7	4.1	4.6	5.2	5.5	5.5	5.6	5.7	3.8	3.5
VII. Diseases of the Circulatory Apparatus	2.1	3.1	2.2	3.0	2.9	3.5	4.2	6.7	5.0	7.3	2.4	3.6
VIII. Diseases of the Respiratory Apparatus	7.5	4.0	8.0	4.1	8.5	3.8	9.7	3.9	10.2	4.7	7.3	3.6
IX. Diseases of the Digestive Apparatus	4.9	5.7	5.0	5.9	6.3	7.5	9.8	11.7	11.8	11.3	5.4	5.8
X. Diseases of the Genitourinary Apparatus	3.1	2.8	3.5	2.7	3.8	2.8	4.6	3.8	4.3	3.8	3.5	3.0
XI. Comp. Related to Pregnancy, Childbirth and the Post-Delivery Period	4.1	12.2	3.5	10.5	3.2	9.8	3.4	8.6	2.1	4.9	6.7	17.3
XII. Diseases of the Skin and the Cellular Tissue under the Skin	3.6	2.2	3.7	2.1	3.5	1.6	3.7	2.5	3.2	1.6	4.5	2.3
XIII. Diseases of the Osteomuscular System and the Connecting Tissue	4.6	4.9	5.8	6.5	6.8	7.6	7.4	6.7	7.2	7.1	4.6	4.8
XIV. Congenital Anomalies	0.1	0.1	0.1	0.1	0.1	0.1	-	-	-	-	-	0.1
XV. Certain Peri. Causes of Morbidity and Mortality	-	-	-	-	-	-	-	-	-	-	-	-
XVI. Badly Defined Symptoms and Diseased States	15.1	14.6	14.4	13.4	14.4	14.3	15.1	13.5	16.5	14.6	11.4	10.4
XVII. Poisoning and Violence	44.6	39.4	43.4	40.7	38.3	36.4	27.0	27.0	22.0	26.2	43.0	37.1
TOTAL	100.0	100.0	100.0	100.0	100.0	100.0	100.0	100.0	100.0	100.0	100.0	100.0

Source: Table 26

TABLE 28: Colombian Social Security Institute: Number of Cases and Days of Incapacity with Subsidies Paid by Age Groups, 1970

Age Group	Cases		Days		Average Number of Days per Case
	Number	(% of total)	Number	(% of total)	
Up to 19 years	5246	3.0	71117	2.6	13.6
20 to 29	39812	22.9	565799	20.6	14.2
30 to 39	37857	21.8	556624	20.3	14.7
40 to 49	17874	10.3	269289	9.8	15.1
50 to 59	7059	4.1	127434	4.6	18.1
60 and over	2532	1.5	64938	2.4	25.6
Age Unspecified	63477	36.5	1087955	39.7	17.1
TOTAL	173857	100.0	2743156	100.0	15.8

Source: Instituto Colombiano de Seguros Sociales, *Estadistica de Casas de Incapacidad Con Subsidio Pagados: Suplemento al Informe Estadistico: Año de 1971* (Bogotá, D.E.: Instituto Colombiano de Seguros Sociales, 1972), pp. 19-21.

TABLE 29: Colombian Social Security Institute: Number of Cases and Days of Incapacity By Economic Sector, 1971

	Cases of Incapacity	Days of Incapacity			
		Illness	Maternity	Work Related Accidents	Total
Primary sector	25153	213130	6171	106772	326073
A. Agriculture, cattle raising, hunting, fishing	22036	191861	5926	90867	288654
B. Extractive Industries	3117	21269	245	15905	37419
Secondary sector	102569	740675	208213	556885	1505773
A. Manufacturing industries	85545	638224	203896	425172	1267292
1. Food industry (except beverages)	13944	113019	28872	63409	205300
2. Beverage industry	4114	27786	3101	20337	51224
3. Tobacco industry	1182	13073	3973	2337	19383
4. Textile industry	10879	85813	34682	42717	163212
5. Footwear, apparel etc. industry	7452	73562	51375	11533	136470
6. Lumber and cork industry	1440	8531	1053	12638	22222
7. Furniture manufacturing	2848	15837	3443	26120	45400
8. Paper, cardboard etc. industry	1580	11887	2340	8130	22357
9. Graphic arts, publicity etc.	2515	24651	9363	8535	42549
10. Manufacture of leather and leather products	1212	9567	3659	5215	18441
11. Manufacture of rubber products	1777	13234	3112	7231	23577
12. Chemical industry and chemical products	4659	37285	16472	22990	76747
13. Industry for petroleum and carbon derivatives	219	1672	196	1758	3626
14. Non-metallic minerals	5489	40771	5834	29579	76184
15. Basic metals industry	5608	27660	2022	40498	70180
16. Metallic products industry	9997	57930	11041	62088	131059
17. Non-electrical machinery industry	2301	13420	981	14265	28666
18. Electrical machinery industry	2884	20801	6732	15724	43257
19. Transportation equipment industry	2562	20615	2602	14559	37776
20. Other manufacturing industries	2883	21110	13043	15509	49662
B. Construction	14511	77435	2180	120244	199859
C. Electricity, gas, steam	2513	25016	2137	11469	38622
Tertiary sector	46135	552861	254637	103812	911310
A. Commerce	21337	258449	100230	41646	400325
1. Wholesale and retail trade	14163	167432	69860	35896	273188
2. Banks and other financial institutions	3369	45109	14976	1851	61936
3. Insurance companies	3071	36039	10517	2286	48842
4. Real estate firms	734	9869	4877	1613	16359
B. Transportation, communication, storage	5336	66288	8535	23690	98453
1. Transportation	4985	63995	8106	19370	91471
2. Warehouses	213	1881	373	1812	4066
3. Communication	165	352	56	2508	2911
C. Services	16435	190011	26646	31175	347832
1. Commercial and social services	8940	113226	59825	15494	188545
2. Recreational services	458	3997	1723	2596	8316
3. Personal services	6780	69339	64757	12508	146604
4. Governmental services	257	3449	341	577	4367
D. Other unclassified	3027	38173	19226	7301	64700
TOTAL	173857	1506666	469021	767469	2743156

Source: Instituto Colombiano de Seguros Sociales, *Estadistica de Casos de Incapacidad con Subsidios Pagados: Suplemento al Informe Estadistico: Año de 1971* (Bogotá, D.E.: Instituto Colombiano de Seguros Sociales, 1972), pp. 13-14.

TABLE 30: Colombian Social Security Institute: Number of Cases and Days of Incapacity by Economic Sector (percentage distribution)

	Cases of Incapacity	Days of Incapacity				Average Total No. of Days per Case
		Illness	Maternity	Work Related Accidents	Total	
I. Primary Sector	14.5	14.1	1.3	13.9	11.9	13
A. Agriculture, cattle raising, hunting, fishing	12.7	12.7	1.3	11.8	10.5	13
B. Extractive industries	1.8	1.4	-	2.1	1.4	12
II. Secondary Sector	59.0	49.2	44.4	72.6	54.9	15
A. Manufacturing industries	49.2	42.4	43.5	55.4	46.2	15
B. Construction	8.3	5.1	0.5	15.7	7.3	14
C. Electricity, gas, steam	1.5	1.7	0.4	1.5	1.4	15
III. Tertiary Sector	26.5	36.7	54.3	13.5	33.2	20
A. Commerce	12.2	17.2	21.4	5.4	14.6	19
B. Transportation, communication, storage	3.1	4.4	1.8	3.1	3.6	18
C. Services	9.5	12.6	27.0	4.0	12.7	21
D. Other	1.7	2.5	4.1	0.9	2.3	21
TOTAL	100.0	100.0	100.0	100.0	100.0	16

Source: Table 29.

affiliated workers, account for about half of all cases of incapacity, 55.4 percent of total days of incapacity due to work-related accidents, and 46.2 percent of total days of incapacity. These tables also reveal that whereas only 5 percent of insured employees work in construction, construction accounts for 8.3 percent of cases of incapacity and 15.7 percent of days of incapacity due to work-related accidents. As a result, the secondary sector represents 59.0 percent of cases of incapacity, 72.6 percent of days of incapacity due to work-related accidents and 54.9 percent of total days of incapacity. The relative share of the primary sector in total cases and days of incapacity is relatively small but larger than the 9 percent of insured employees in this sector. On the other hand, the tertiary sector, which includes 44 percent of insured employees, represents only 26.5 percent total cases and 33.2 percent of total days of incapacity. However, this sector represents over half of days of incapacity due to maternity, presumably due to the relatively larger proportion of women employed in commerce and the provision of personal services.

Willingness-to-Pay estimates

The distribution of benefits from health services by income class estimated on a willingness-to-pay basis is presented in Table 24. Health services provided by ICSS generate private use-of-income benefits for recipients. These benefits were imputed by income class using the general functional form for the marginal utility of income proposed by Maital in order to apply the Aaron and McGuire Theorem and an elasticity of marginal utility with respect to income equal to one. As stated in Chapter 1, this treatment of all publicly provided health services was defended by Neenan with the argument that whereas the consumer is free to adjust the quantity consumed in the private sector, if his income increases and/or he wishes to consume more, he is not free to adjust the quantity of the public good consumed; the quantity of health services provided by the public sector is fixed.[70]

The incidence, on the willingness-to-pay basis, is proportional over all income classes, with benefits equal to 6.3 percent of income.[71] Benefits per worker were found to increase continuously as income increased. Finally, whereas the two lowest income classes were imputed about 21 percent of total benefits, when benefits were estimated on a cost-of-service basis, they were imputed only 8 percent, when benefits were estimated on a willingness-to-pay basis.

TABLE 31: Colombian Social Security Institute: Net Fiscal Residuals — Benefits Estimated on a Cost-of-Service Basis and on a Willingness-to-Pay Basis

Income Bracket (Pesos per year)	Benefits (Cost of Service Basis) (millions of pesos)	Social Security Taxes (millions of pesos)	Net Fiscal Residuals (Millions of pesos)	Net Fiscal Residuals (% of income)	Net Fiscal Residuals (pesos per worker)	Benefits Willingness-to-pay-Basis) (millions of pesos)	Social Security Taxes (millions of pesos)	Net Fiscal Residuals (millions of pesos)	Net Fiscal Residuals (% of income)	Net Fiscal Residuals (pesos per worker)
0-4,319.99	31.1	10.7	20.4	15.1	+544.0	8.5	10.7	-2.2	-1.6	- 58.7
4,320-6,479.99	155.4	33.3	122.1	12.4	+672.0	62.1	33.3	28.8	2.9	+158.5
6,480-9,359.99	212.2	64.5	147.7	9.0	+714.2	103.0	64.5	38.5	2.4	+186.2
9,360-12,959.99	166.9	68.3	98.6	5.7	+638.2	108.3	68.3	40.0	2.3	+258.9
12,960-17,999.99	137.6	83.2	54.4	2.7	+421.7	126.1	83.2	42.9	2.1	+332.6
18,000-24,479.99	99.4	95.8	3.6	0.2	+ 34.3	140.2	95.8	44.4	2.0	+422.9
24,480-33,839.99	45.3	82.2	- 36.9	- 2.5	- 719.3	94.1	82.2	11.9	0.8	+232.0
33,840-45,359.99	19.5	73.4	- 53.9	- 4.6	1833.3	73.7	73.4	0.3	-	+ 10.2
45,360-60,479.99	10.7	63.4	- 52.7	- 5.0	-2661.6	66.6	63.4	3.2	0.3	+161.6
60,480 and over	9.8	278.8	-269.0	-16.1	-10590.6	104.8	278.8	-174.0	-10.4	+6850.4
TOTAL	887.8	853.6				887.8	853.6			

Sources: Tables 23, 24.

NET FISCAL INCIDENCE OF HEALTH EXPENDITURES OF THE COLOMBIAN SOCIAL SECURITY INSTITUTE BY INCOME CLASS, 1970

Table 31 presents two sets of net fiscal residuals, one calculated on the basis of cost-of-service estimates of benefits and the estimated distribution of taxes and the other calculated on the basis of willingness-to-pay estimates of benefits and the same distribution of taxes. The former were found to be largest for the second and third income classes from the bottom and negative for those in the four highest income classes, or those above the 24,480 pesos per annum income level. The same was true for net fiscal residuals per worker. In addition, residuals as a percentage of income were found to decline monotonically over all income classes. Hence, the incidence may be described as regressive, or pro-poor.

Fiscal residuals estimated on the basis of willingness-to-pay estimates of benefits and the estimated distribution of taxes were found to be largest for those in the fourth, fifth, and sixth income classes from the bottom, or those more or less in the middle income classes, and negative for those in either the lowest or the highest income group; fiscal residuals per worker provided similar results. The incidence pattern was found to be progressive (pro-rich) at the bottom of the scale, approximately proportional with a hint of regressivity in moving from the second income class to the sixth income class from the bottom, and then sharply regressive in moving over the remaining income classes at the top of the scale.[72]

Summary

The purpose of this chapter was to apply the theoretical analysis contained in Chapters 1 and 2 in an empirical analysis of the redistributive effects of public health expenditures in Colombia. The chapter consisted of two parts. The first contained an analysis of the incidence of expenditures of the Ministry of Public Health in 1970, the incidence of taxes collected by the Central Government, which are used to finance these expenditures, and an analysis of the net fiscal incidence of these government activities; the second part consisted of an analysis of the incidence of health expenditures of the Colombian Social Security Institute in 1970, the incidence of social security contributions and small additional revenues, and the net fiscal incidence of these government activities. The procedures adopted and the results of the analysis are summarized below for each of these two institutions.

The Ministry of Public Health

The analysis regarding the Ministry of Public Health proceeded by first estimating the underlying distribution of income among Colombian households in urban and rural areas and among households in the nation as a whole in 1970, using various surveys conducted by the national statistics office, DANE. The results indicated that the distribution of income is highly unequal; the bottom 45 percent of all households only receives about 14 percent of total income, while the top 13 percent receives about 50 percent of total income. Furthermore, several adjustments were made to these income data for the purpose of estimating tax incidence. These are referred to below.

Tax collections of the central government were then allocated by income class using standard incidence assumptions. Direct taxes were allocated as follows: (1) personal income taxes were allocated by income class using unpublished tax return data for 1967, which were adjusted to the year 1970 and to allow for the ceding of income between husband and wife; (2) the corporation income tax was allocated under three alternative assumptions: (A) that the tax is borne by Colombian shareholders, who were assumed to be in the 3 highest income brackets; (B) that it is borne by Colombian consumers, and was therefore allocated in proportion to the distribution of non-food consumption expenditures by income class, according to a DANE household expenditure survey for urban areas in 1970; and (C) that it is borne by non-Colombian shareholders; (3) coffee export duties were allocated using data on the size of plantings and the value of coffee production. In the analysis of the corporation income tax, in case (A), income data were adjusted for retained earnings and the unshifted portion of the corporation income tax on the assumption that the former enhances the economic position of shareholders and that incomes would have been higher by an amount equal to the tax, if it had not been imposed; in case (B), income data were adjusted for retained earnings. The rural income distribution was adjusted for the amount of coffee export duties attributed to each income level on the assumption that incomes would have been higher by this amount, if the tax had not been imposed.

In allocating indirect taxes by income class, the following procedures were employed: (1) gasoline taxes were allocated on the basis of estimated use of motor fuel by private automobile users, municipal buses, intermunicipal buses, and cargo carriers; the 1970 DANE household consumption survey for urban areas provided relevant consumption data by income class which were used as allocative guides; (2) customs duties and (3) stamp taxes were allocated on the basis of the distribution of non-food consumption expenditures by income class; and (4) revenue collected under the 4 rates of the national sales tax was allocated on the basis of non-food consumption expenditures (3 percent rate); consumption of tobacco products (10 percent rate); and automobile purchases (8 and 15 percent rates).

The results of these allocative procedures and the estimated effective tax rates for all taxes are summarized in Tables 11 and 12. The overall tax system was found to be progressive, but the degree of progressivity varied from mild to fairly strong, depending upon whether the corporation income tax is assumed to have been borne by upper income Colombian shareholders, by Colombian consumers, or by foreigners. Furthermore, the personal income tax was found to be an important factor contributing to the overall progressivity of the system.

Health expenditures of the Ministry of Public Health were then analyzed using the standard cost-of-service methodology and using the conceptually preferable willingness-to-pay methodology. Total expenditures of the Ministry were grouped into the following categories: maternal/child care, rural sanitation, urban sanitation, medical-hospital care, epidemiology, and other expenditures. In making cost-of-service estimates, benefits were allocated to beneficiaries on the basis of user data, in the cases of maternal/child care and medical-hospital care, and under the assumption that benefits were provided to all households in a given benefit area, that is, to rural households in the case of rural sanitation, to urban households in the case of urban sanitation, and to all households in the case of epidemiology. Other, mainly administrative, expenditures were allocated by income class in proportion to the distribution, by income class, of those expenditures classified as Public Health by the Ministry. In making estimates using the willingness-to-pay methodology, benefits were not only imputed to direct beneficiaries of redistributive programs, such as maternal/child care, but also to non-recipient taxpayers who were "willing-to-pay" for these services. Hence, source-of-income benefits were imputed to recipients of maternal/child care services and use-of-income benefits were imputed to upper income taxpayers; private, use-of-income benefits were attributed to income classes that were estimated to benefit from medical-hospital care; public nonredistributive, use-of-income benefits were imputed to all income classes in a given benefit area, as in the case of cost-of-service estimates, in allocating the benefits of rural and urban sanitation and epidemiology; and other expenditures were imputed on the basis of the distribution of benefits from services classified under Public Health. However, in imputing use-of-income benefits across income classes, it was assumed that the elasticity of marginal utility with respect to income equals one, whereas in making cost-of-service estimates, it is implicitly assumed to be zero.

The results of these allocative assumptions are summarized in Tables 13 and 14. The incidence of benefits based upon the cost-of-service methodology was significantly more pro-poor or regressive than the incidence of benefits based on the willingness-to-pay methodology. The cost-of-service estimates may be regarded as defining the most pro-poor benefit incidence pattern, or the extreme case. The less regressive benefit incidence pattern which emerged from the willingness-to-pay estimates is attributable to two important assumptions, namely that the marginal utility of income declines proportionately to income and that some health expenditures, such as those for maternal/child care, also generate public benefits.

The two patterns of net fiscal residuals presented in Tables 15 and 16 reflect the combined effect of the progressivity of the tax system and the pro-poor distribution of benefits from health services provided by the Ministry of Health according to each of the two sets of benefit estimates, respectively. Under both patterns, the two lower income classes enjoy positive residuals, while upper income groups were estimated to have negative residuals; however, residuals for lower income groups are less favorable and those for upper income groups are less adverse when benefits are estimated on a willingness-to-pay basis.

The Colombian Social Securtiy Institute

The Colombian Social Security Institute provides health services mainly to workers employed in private manufacturing industries through a compulsory system of health insurance. The largest proportion of these workers (42 percent) are in the 4,320 to 9,360 pesos per year or 360 to 780 pesos per month, income range (See Table 18.) Health services are primarily financed by compulsory social security payroll taxes, which are shared by the employer and the employee. These were allocated by income class using the statutory rates that applied in 1970 and on the assumption that the employee's and half of the employer's share are borne by the employee, while the other half of the employer's share is shifted to consumers and was therefore allocated on the basis of total consumption expenditures by income class. Health services in poor areas are subsidized through transfers from the central government into the Solidarity Fund, and these were allocated in proportion to the distribution of national taxes. The results of these allocative procedures are summarized in Table 23. They indicate that the incidence of social security contributions, including the small amount of national taxes transferred by the Central Government into the Solidarity Fund, is mildly progressive over most income classes but strongly progressive at the top of the scale mainly due to the use of consumption expenditures in the allocative procedure.

Benefits from health services provided by the Colombian Social Security Institute were also allocated by income class using the cost-of-service and the willingness-to-pay methodologies. In the former case, the distribution of patients by income class who had received subsidies while unable to work was used as an allocative guide. In the latter case, it was assumed that private, use-of-income benefits were generated for all income classes and that the marginal utility of income declines proportionately to income. The empirical results, which are summarized in Table 24, indicate that benefit incidence is regressive when benefits are estimated on a cost-of-service basis and proportional when estimated on a willingness-to-pay basis. This variation in the benefit incidence patterns is reflected in the two patterns of net fiscal residuals presented in Table 31. They indicate that the largest fiscal residuals are not estimated for the second and third income classes from the bottom, or for those in the 4,320 to 9,360 income range, as cost-of-service estimates indicate, but rather for the fifth and sixth income classes, or for those in the 12,960 to 24,480 income range.

NOTES AND REFERENCES

[1] The Urban Institute, "Unscrambling Metropolitan Fiscal Flows," *Search: A Report from the Urban Institute* 4 (January-April 1974):5.

[2] The equiproportional tax-allocation assumption has generated some discussion in the literature. See, for example, W. Lee Hansen and Burton A. Weisbrod, "The Distribution of Costs and Benefits of Public Higher Education: The Case of California," *The Journal of Human Resources* 4 (Spring 1969): 176-91; Joseph A. Pechman, "The Distributional Effects of Public Higher Education in California," *The Journal of Human Resources* 5 (Summer 1970): 361-70; Robert W. Hartman, "A Comment on the Pechman-Hansen-Weisbrod Controversy," *The Journal of Human Resources* 5 (Fall 1970): 519-23; W. Lee Hansen and Burton A. Weisbrod, "Who Pays for a Public Expenditure Program?" *National Tax Journal* 24 (December 1971): 515-17.

[3] These surveys are described in Polibio Córdova, *La Encuesta Nacional de Hogares de Colombia* (Bogotá, D.E.: Departamento Administrativo Nacional de Estadistica [DANE], 1971). Data for the distribution of income in rural areas are from Project EH-1 and these are presented in Polibio Córdova, *Distribución de Ingresos en Colombia* (Bogotá, D.E.: Departamento Administrativo Nacional de Estadistico [DANE], 1971). DANE provided data from Project EH-2 for the distribution of income in urban areas in unpublished form to McLure.

[4] Charles E. McLure, Jr., "The Incidence of Colombian Taxes, 1970," Paper No. 41, William Marsh Rice University, Houston, Texas, Summer 1973, pp. 3-13.

[5] Córdoba, *Distribucion de Ingresos en Colombia*, p. 61, quoted in Spanish by McLure, "The Incidence of Colombian Taxes, 1970," p. 3.

[6] Polibio Córdova, "Agregación de Municipios a las Ciudades Investigadas in la Segunda Etapa de Encuesta de Hogares y Cálculo de Factores de Expansión." This memorandum describes a suggested assignment of regions to representative cities and the calculation of the number of households in each region.

[7] Córdova, *Distribucion de Ingresos en Colombia*, pp. 80, 84, and 95; and McLure, "The Incidence of Colombian Taxes, 1970," p. 8.

[8] This distribution is significantly less unequal than the distribution of agricultural income in 1960 estimated by Berry and Padilla and the distribution of rural income in 1964 estimated by Urrutia. Agricultural income accruing to urban persons was included in both of those studies, whereas McLure excluded it, and this in part may explain the discrepancy. See Albert Berry and Alfonso Padilla, "La Distribucion de Ingresos Provenientes de la Agricultura en Colombia—1960," *Boletin Mensual de Estadistica* (DANE, January 1971), ppl xxi-xxvi; and Miguel Urrutia, "La Distribucion de Ingresos en Colombia," (Bogotá: Banco de la Republica). (Xeroxed.) Cited by McLure, "The Incidence of Colombian Taxes," *op. cit.*, p. 10.

[9] McLure, "The Incidence of Colombian Taxes, *op. cit.*, p. 12.

[10] *Ibid.*, pp. 12-13.

[11] *Ibid.*, pp. 14-16.

[12] *Ibid.*, pp. 16-17.

[13] *Ibid.*, p. 14.

[14] This part of the study relies heavily upon *Ibid.*, pp. 21-61.

[15] For a discussion of the possible use of alternative assumptions see: R. A. Musgrave, J. J. Carroll, L. D. Cook, and L. Frane, "Distribution of Tax Payments by Income Groups: A Case Study for 1948," *National Tax Journal* 4 (March 1951): 14.

[16] McLure, "The Incidence of Colombian Taxes, 1970," pp. 23-25, 58-61. (In 1970, a husband could cede one-half of his labor income to his wife, but this amount could not exceed 30,000 pesos per year.)

[17] Only includes coffee export duties paid to the Central Government.

[18] Actual collections of indirect taxes in 1969 were used, as only budget estimates were available for 1970.

[19] The amount of the petroleum subsidy implicit in the differential petroleum exchange rate was subtracted from gasoline tax collections.

[20] This information was only available for machine-processes income tax returns; they were used to estimate the net amounts ceded to or from income classes on all tax returns by applying the ratio of total income in each income class to the income recorded on machine-processed returns.

[21] McLure, "The Incidence of Colombian Taxes," *op. cit.*, p. 24.

[22] *Ibid.*, pp. 25-26.

[23] *Ibid.*, p. 27.

[24] The possibility that a significant portion of the tax is shifted to non-Colombian consumers was not considered very likely and was therefore disregarded.

[25] It could also have been assumed that the tax is shifted to consumers and retained earnings could have been allocated to foreigners. However, this combination was not included as a fourth alternative because the results would not have differed qualitatively from those estimated under alternative (B). See McLure, "The Incidence of Colombian Taxes," *op. cit.*, p. 15.

[26] *Ibid.*, p. 32.

[27] *Ibid.*

[28] *Ibid.*, p. 17.

[29] McLure adopted polar assumptions in analyzing the incidence of coffee export duties. One set of estimates is based on the assumption that all coffee duties are truly taxes on the coffee sector and the other set of estimates is based on the assumption that none are, i.e. that these revenues flow back into the coffee sector. In fact, however, the Central Government receives most of the coffee export tax, but the remainder of this tax, the pasilla, and the retention tax are returned to the National Coffee Fund, as indicated above.

[30] *Ibid.*, pp. 17-20.

[31] McLure estimated effective tax rates for the rural sector of 6.3 and 59.3 percent for the lowest and the highest income levels, respectively. See *Ibid.*, p. 34.

[32] *Ibid.*, pp. 42-44, 49.

[33]The operation of the differential exchange rate is discussed in: Gillis and Musgrave, (eds.), *Fiscal Reform for Colombia: The Final Report and Staff Papers of the Colombian Commission on Tax Reform*, pp. 692-719.

[34]*Ibid.*, pp. 45-49.

[35]*Ibid.*

[36]See pp. 48-50, 93-94.

[37]Alcides Estrada, "Caracteristicas de las Mujeres que Solicitaron el Servicio de Planificacion Familiar en el Programa Materno Infantil del Ministerio de Salud Publica—Estadisticas de Servicio Primer Semestre de 1973," paper prepared for the Ministerio de Salud Publica and the Centro Regional de Poblacion, Bogotá, D.E., December 1973, p. 7. (Mimeographed.)

[38]Departamento Administrativo Nacional de Estadistica (Dane), "Estructura del consumo relacionado con la salud," *boletin mensual de estadistica* 264-265 (July-August 1973): 32-38.

[39]Some interpolations were required, as the income brackets did not coincide with those of the income distribution data.

[40]The expenditure data available did not permit a more detailed analysis of the distribution of the benefits of particular health services, such as inpatient and outpatient care, by income class.

[41]See p. 41.

[42]See p. 110.

[43]The incidence of health benefits measured on a willingness-to-pay basis was also found to be pro-poor over most income classes both when the elasticity of marginal utility with respect to income was assumed to be 1.5 and 2.0.

[44]Buchanan was the first to employ the term fiscal residual to describe the net incidence of taxes and expenditures on individuals. He indicated the need to apply the principle of horizontal equity to the net impact of the budget rather than to tax incidence alone. If the excess of benefits from public expenditures over taxes paid is equalized among equals, then the principle of horizontal equity is being implemented. See Greene, Neenan, and Scott, *Fiscal Interactions in a Metropolitan Area*, *op. cit.*, p. 157.

[45]Residuals as a percentage of money income were also found to decline monotonically over all income classes when elasticities of marginal utility with respect to income of 1.5 and 2.0 were assumed.

[46]Milton Friedman, "Transfer Payments and the Social Security System," *The Conference Room* (New York: Columbia University Press, 1965), pp. 11, 7-10.

[47]George Jaszi, "A Critique of the United States Income and Product Accounts," *Studies in Income and Wealth*, vol. 22 (Prince-

ton: National Bureau of Economic Research, 1958), pp. 400-430.

[48] Harold M. Groves, *Financing Government*, 3d ed., (New York: Henry Holt and Company, Inc., 1951).

[49] Groves, *Financing Government*, p. 157, quoted in John A. Brittain, "The Incidence of Social Security Payroll Taxes," *The American Economic Review* 61 (March 1971): 111.

[50] *Ibid.*, pp. 113-24. and ________, *The Payroll Tax for Social Security* (Washington, D.C.: The Brookings Institution, 1972), pp. 60-81.

[51] He qualifies the reasoning summarized above in two ways: (1) In emphasizing real factor shares, the actual mechanism of the shifting process is not discussed; backward shifting via a money wage effect, and forward shifting, via a price effect, are not distinguished; (2) The probably numerous microeconomic effects of social security taxes due to different rates and elasticities are ignored. See *Ibid.*, p. 115.

[52] *Ibid.*

[53] *Ibid.*

[54] Martin S. Feldstein, "The Incidence of the Social Security Payroll Tax: Comment," *The American Economic Review* 62 (September 1972): 735-36.

[55] Brittain, "Social Security Payroll Taxes," *op. cit.*, p. 122.

[56] Feldstein, "Social Security Payroll Tax: Comment," *op. cit.*, pp. 735-42.

[57] *Ibid.*, p. 736.

[58] *Ibid.*, p. 738. In a more recent econometric study of the U.S. social security system, Feldstein found that social security reduces personal saving by 30-50 percent and reduces the capital stock and the level of national income. He argues that the net effect of the reduction in the capital stock due to the social security program lowers wage rates and raises the rate of profit. See Martin Feldstein, "Social Security, Induced Retirement, and Aggregate Capital Accumulation," *Journal of Political Economy* 82 (September/October 1974): 923-25.

[59] John A. Brittain, "The Incidence of the Social Security Payroll Tax: Reply," *The American Economic Review* 62 (September 1972): 739; See also *Ibid.*, pp. 739-42.

[60] *Ibid.*, p. 742.

[61] Gillespie, *The Incidence of Taxes*, *op. cit.*, pp. 55-56.

[62] See pp. 124-25.

[63] Instituto Colombiano de Seguros Sociales, *Informe del Director General: 1.970-1.971*, p. 88.

[64] Instituto Colombiano de Seguros Sociales, *Informe Estadistico: 1971*, p. 33.

[65] See pp. 107, 112.

[66] See pp. 103-104.

[67] See p. 109.

[68] McLure, "On the Theory and Methodology," *op. cit.*, p. 65.

[69] De Wulf, "Fiscal Incidence Studies," *op. cit.*, pp. 44-45.

[70] See p. 40.

[71] The incidence of health benefits on a willingness-to-pay basis was found to be progressive (pro-rich), however, when elasticities of marginal utility with respect to income of 1.5 and 2.0 were assumed.

[72] When an elasticity of marginal utility with respect to income of 1.5 was assumed, the incidence pattern was found to be progressive (pro-rich), over all income classes, but regressive in moving from the tenth to the eleventh income class from the bottom; the estimated incidence pattern was, of course, even more progressive over all income classes, with the exception of the slight regressivity at the top of the scale, when an elasticity of marginal utility with respect to income of 2.0 was assumed.

Chapter 5

SUMMARY AND CONCLUSIONS

General Introduction

In this chapter the redistributive impact of public health expenditures in Colombia on the size distribution of income is summarized for the two institutions studied, the Colombian Social Security Institute (ICSS) and the Ministry of Public Health. In the light of these estimates, a number of relevant theoretical, empirical, and policy issues will be discussed. In particular, the chapter includes: (1) a brief summary of the empirical results with respect to benefit, tax, and net fiscal incidence, including an attempt to highlight the practical consequences of the two methodologies employed; (2) a discussion of the future of health policy in Colombia in relation to these results and more recent developments in the health sector; (3) a discussion of how a higher level of health expenditures may be financed; and (4) a summary of the limitations of both the data and the methodology.

Summary of Empirical Results

A comparison of the incidence pattern that emerges according to each of the two approaches employed in this study may serve to point out the practical importance of some of the issues discussed in Chapters 1 and 2. The *benefit incidence* analysis shows that: (1) the poor enjoy significantly "higher" benefits if the cost-of-service approach is used to allocate benefits than when benefits are allocated using the willingness-to-pay approach, and this was found to be true of the results for both ICSS and the Ministry of Public Health (See Chapter 4, Tables 13, 14, and 24.); when benefits are allocated under the willingness-to-pay procedure, estimated benefit incidence for the poor is reduced while that for higher income households is increased relative to the cost-of-service estimates; (2) under the cost-of-service approach, benefits relative to income decline monotonically over all income classes in the cases of both ICSS and the Ministry of Public Health; using the willingness-to-pay approach, benefits relative to income are found to be proportional over all income classes in the case of ICSS and to be regressive over the three lowest income groups and from the fourth to the fifth income group from the bottom and approximately proportional over the three highest income classes in the case of the Ministry of Public Health.

Tax incidence estimated for taxes levied by the national government and for taxes levied by ICSS is found to be progressive (See Chapter 4, Tables 11, 12, 22, and 23.) The overall progressivity of National taxes is found to range from mild to fairly strong, depending upon whether the corporate income tax is borne by Colombian consumers or foreigners or by Colombian shareholders. The incidence of social security taxes is found to be slightly progressive over most income groups but strongly progressive at the top of the scale, reflecting the allocation of employer contributions in proportion to consumption expenditure in urban areas.

Combining the analysis of tax and benefit incidence, *fiscal residuals* were derived from willingness-to-pay estimates of benefits and from cost-of-service estimates of benefits (See Chapter 4, Tables 15, 16, and 31.) The residual pattern derived from cost-of-service estimates is regressive in relation to income for both the Ministry of Public Health, under both assumptions A and B, and ICSS; in relation to income, the largest positive fiscal residual confronts the lowest income group and residuals decline monotonically over all income classes. In the case of the Ministry of Public Health, the residual pattern derived from willingness-to-pay estimates of benefits is also regressive in relation to income under both assumptions, but less regressive than in the case of cost-of-service estimates; the largest positive fiscal residual, in relation to income, also confronts the lowest income group. Residuals derived from willingness-to-pay estimates of benefits for ICSS indicate a negative residual for the lowest income group and substantially smaller positive fiscal residuals for lower income groups than residuals estimated using cost-of-service benefits indicate. On the other hand, fiscal residuals for upper income groups are more favorable or less negative as income increases.

Data pertaining directly to citizen attitudes toward public health programs in Colombia unfortunately are not available. However, some of the results obtained using the willingness-to-pay estimates appear compatible with those of the Frey and Kohn analysis of eighteen public finance referenda in Basel-Stadt Switzerland, where tax incidence also is progressive.[1] Frey and Kohn found voter support to be highest in the lowest income group, lower in the next highest group and then more or less constant across income classes. Fiscal residuals estimated for middle and upper income beneficiaries of services provided by the Ministry of Public Health under assumption B appear to reflect a similar pattern. As previous empirical studies indicate, however, the willingness-to-pay for expenditure programs varies not only with attitudes toward programs but also with anticipated tax liability.[2] Furthermore, since these fiscal residuals reflect the average of all estimated health benefits and all national taxes, in the analysis of the Ministry of Public Health services, the pattern of support for any one program need not have the same shape.

In conclusion, the benefit incidence pattern and the pattern of net fiscal residuals estimated using the willingness-to-pay approach suggest that public health benefits are not distributed as regressively (that is, as pro-poor) as suggested by results obtained under the standard methodology used in previous studies, namely the cost-of-service approach. This suggests that it would take greater progressivity of the tax-transfer system to achieve the redistribution desired and in fact suggested as being achieved by estimates derived using the standard methodology.

The Future of Health Policy in Colombia

The empirical results indicate that public health services are designed to achieve Colombia's objective of reducing the gap in health status between the rich and the poor, as part of an overall strategy for improving the distribution of income. Nevertheless, the government is aware of deficiencies in the health care system, and since 1971, Colombia has taken further measures to directly increase and improve health services available to the poor. This study encompassed expenditure for health services and taxes in fiscal 1970 and many of the health programs emphasized in subsequent phases of the National Health Plan are primarily extensions of successful programs already in existence in 1970.

The empirical analysis in Chapter 4 indicates that the single most important health program *specifically* directed at the vast majority of the poorest strata of the Colombian population is that for mothers and children. The benefits of maternal/child care services are concentrated in the two lowest income groups. Of total benefits from programs of the Ministry of Public Health allocated to this group, these represent over two-thirds on a willingness-to-pay basis and over half on a cost-of-service basis. As mentioned in Chapter 3, the maternal/child care program includes pre-natal, obstetric, and post-partum attention, well-child clinics, attention to diseases particularly affecting children and mothers, family planning services, general hygiene and nutrition education, and supplementary food programs. Children under 15 and fecund women constitute about 70 percent of the total population, as was also pointed out in Chapter 3. Morbidity and mortality rates are high among these lower income groups, as they are unable to purchase an adequate diet or adequate health services and because they live and raise large families under poor unsanitary conditions. These services need to be expanded and the government has given high priority to expanding them, particularly in rural areas. Using auxiliary personnel, particularly *promotoras* and auxiliary nurses, the authorities have been increasing the accessibility of health services to children and mothers in rural areas and in urban areas without adequate access to health care.[3]

Empirical results indicate that the second most important health program for the poor is rural sanitation. The two lowest income groups receive over three-fourths of the benefits from this program on a cost-of-service basis and over two-fifths on a willingness-to-pay basis. While curative health care systems mainly reduce the effects of diseases, better water supply and sewerage services can contribute to reducing the "incidence" of a larger number of diseases affecting the poorest segments of the population. Colombia's efficiently managed INPES program has expanded rapidly. It provided rural aqueducts to 695,629 inhabitants of rural population centers of 50 to 2,500 people from August 1970 to June 1974, compared to 660,635 inhabitants during the period 1961 to July 1970.[4] Nevertheless, in June 1974 only 52.5 percent of the rural population living in rural localities had been covered. The deficit is even larger in regard to rural sewerage systems. INPES provided sewerage facilities to 150,658 people during the period August 1970 to June 1974, compared to 227,064 people from 1961 to June 1970, but in June 1974, only 14.8 percent of the rural population living in communities had been covered.[5]

Lower income groups share relatively less in benefits from general medical-hospital services than in benefits from maternal-child care and rural sanitation programs. The two lowest income groups were estimated to receive only 17 percent of benefits from these services on a cost-of-service basis and 16 percent on a willingness-to-pay basis. Those in the third and fourth income classes from the bottom benefit most. Low utilization rates by the poor need to be increased. The latter could be achieved by improving the quality of services, providing them in convenient locations, influencing cultural attitudes and practices through outreach programs using para-medical personnel and by levying charges, discussed further below, that do not discourage utilization by low income groups. Furthermore, the cost of providing medical care needs to be reduced.

In recent years the government has been expanding and improving curative health services in rural and urban areas, while attempting to reduce costs by limiting substantial capital expenditures on sophisticated hospital facilities. This has entailed reorganizing the public health system into a regionalized integrated health system.[6] The "regionalization" concept refers to the referral of patients between the different levels of the pyramid of institutions which provide health care: health post, health center, local hospital, regional hospital, and university hospital. Emphasis is on expanding health posts and health centers, increased utilization of auxiliary personnel, particularly *promotoras* and auxiliary nurses, developing an effective patient referral system between lower and more sophisticated levels of care, and greater use of out-patient care. Simultaneously, the government is attempting to integrate preventive health services, such as environmental sanitation programs, malaria and other endemic disease control programs, carried out more or less independently through various institutions and programs, into the regionalized system.

Expenditures on nationwide campaigns against epidemic diseases, including nationwide campaigns against smallpox, tuberculosis, diphtheria, whooping cough, polio, measles, malaria, yellow fever and yaws, and expenditures on urban sanitation appear to directly benefit the poor to an even lesser extent than medical-hospital care, when benefits are allocated on a willingness to pay basis. The two lowest income groups were allocated eight percent and three percent of benefits generated by campaigns against epidemic diseases and urban sanitation services, respectively, using the willingness-to-pay approach (39 percent and 15 percent, respectively, using the cost-of-service approach).

Little empirical work has been done on the appropriate mix of health services. According to the willingness-to-pay estimates in this study, discussed above, relatively small proportions of the benefits from national campaigns against epidemic diseases, urban sanitation services, and general medical-hospital care were allocated to the poor. Providing adequate sanitation services entails the investment of substantial financial resources in infrastructure. However, these contribute to reducing the incidence of a wide range of diseases, while curative health care, as mentioned earlier, only lessens the effects of diseases. Furthermore, as migration of the poor to urban areas continues, their share of the benefits from urban sanitation services may be expected to increase.

Empirical analysis of medical care provided by ICSS indicates that about one-third of benefits estimated on a willingness-to-pay basis accrues to recipients with an annual income of less than 13,000 pesos. However, cost-of-service estimates of benefits based on user data reveal that these individuals receive an estimated 64 percent of benefits. Consequently, on the basis of user data, it does not appear that: "In the case of ICSS, . . . the main beneficiaries are families in the middle and upper-middle income ranges."[7] Utilization rates by lower income groups appear to be high, in contrast to rates among lower income households served by medical care facilities of the Ministry of Public Health. This may be due to a number of factors, including the quality of service and the absence of direct charges for services rendered. These services could be provided to a larger proportion of the poorer strata of society by extending coverage to spouse and children, if they are not salaried, and also to the self-employed in urban and rural areas. Coverage is now limited to insured male and female employees, the wife of an insured employee in the case of pregnancy, and the child during its first twelve months of life.[8] If the population covered by ICSS is expanded and Ministry of Public Health responsibility for curative health care is reduced, the Ministry could devote a larger share of its financial resources to preventive measures.

Financing a Higher Level of Public Health Expenditures

Colombian authorities implemented major changes in the national tax system in the last four mounths of 1974. The reform was based upon, and in a number of cases improved upon, proposals by the 1968-69 Colombian Commission on Tax Reform, known as the Musgrave Commission.[9] Among the principal objectives of the tax reform were the achievement of greater progressivity in the distribution of the tax burden and greater revenue yield. To improve the progressivity of the tax system, the authorities adjusted the rate structure of the personal income tax; eliminated many deductions and exempt income items, mainly benefiting upper income groups, and converted most of the remaining exemptions and deductions into tax credits, the benefits of which do not increase as a taxpayer's marginal tax rate increases; adjusted the rate structure of the net wealth tax and eliminated numerous exemptions which existed under the former law; limited the scope for tax avoidance and evasion by recipients of capital income, who are primarily located in upper income groups, by introducing a new tax on irregular income; substantially revised death and gift taxes; and made many services consumed primarily by upper income groups subject to the sales tax for the first time. The reform also included many other measures designed to improve resource allocation and to facilitate tax administration and reduce the scope for tax evasion.

Legally, a substantial share of any increase in government revenue must be allocated for education and health services. Since 1973, a share of central government revenue is required to be transferred to departments, *intendencias*, *comisarias*, and the Special District of Bogota. They must use the funds to finance current expenditures on health and primary education. This revenue sharing scheme is known as the *situado fiscal*. According to the law, the share was to increase from a minimum of 13 percent in 1973, to 14 percent in 1974, 15 percent in 1975 and thereafter by two percentage points per year until a maximum of 25 percent is attained, provided that ordinary revenue rises at a minimum average rate of 15 percent over the three preceding years. Each recipient must spend 74 percent of the funds received for primary education and 26 percent for public health; 20 percent of the amount transferred is apportioned equally among recipients, the "Situado Fiscal Territorial," and 70 percent on the basis of population, the "Situado Fiscal de Poblacion." To ensure that the recipient will increase expenditures on primary education and health, each unit is required to appropriate a percentage of its own revenues, apart from the transfers, for primary education and public health equal to or exceeding the percentage allocated for these services in 1972. In the case of public health, these funds are transferred to the Sectional Health Services.[10]

As government finances improve, the level of expenditure on other health related services may also be expected to increase and a greater share of these services could be financed through general tax revenue than through direct charges for these services. In Colombia, price discrimination, particularly for hospital services, appears to be widespread, with charges varying according to the recipient's ability to pay. While the level of charges should not discourage utilization by low income groups, retaining charges for health services may be justified not only because they are a source of income for institutions providing the services but also to discourage malingering and perhaps also because people may only appreciate what they are required to pay for. For example, in Germany, which has had compulsory health insurance through the social security system since 1883, patients make no direct payments. As a result, demand for medical attention is almost limitless and the physician's time is frequently wasted treating trivial problems not warranting his attention.

Some have concluded, therefore, that:

> . . . the introduction of direct cost sharing by the patient for all items of medical care is the only way to eliminate a major part of the abuses and absurdities which have developed under our present system. Every patient should pay directly a share of the doctor's bill, the prescriptions as well as hospitalization. Exceptions might be made for certain very low-income groups, and there is some justification for letting the compulsory agencies assume complete financial responsibility for certain long and very severe ailments, after an initial period of cost sharing by the patient. But in all other cases, it seems absolutely necessary to make the patient share the cost to an extent which will allow him to think twice before incurring the expense. This is the only way to make clear to the sick person the value of medical services. Not only the status of the physician but very probably his therapeutic effectiveness as well have suffered in many cases from the fact that the patient has not the remotest idea of the value of his treatment in monetary terms. Cost sharing has the advantage that even without a complicated supervision and control system, the patient himself carefully keeps track of the services actually rendered to him. Naturally he will refuse to pay for medical care which was not given him. And, finally, the doctors will only be freed from the burden of trivial cases if medical care costs something to those who seek it.[11]

However, reforming the German system has proven politically difficult. The British government has been able to introduce more and more direct charges for specific services to finance the National Health Service. The system, nevertheless, has many shortcomings. Furthermore, the payment is refunded if the patient persuades the authorities that it would constitute an undue hardship.[12]

Medical care provided by ICSS has been adversely affected by inadequate financial resources. One-fourth of contributions were to have been provided by the government, one-fourth by the employee, and the remainder by the employer. In practice, the government has not complied with this requirement. Since 1973, the government has agreed to contribute one-fourth of actual expenditures by ICSS for medical care, but it has not complied with this either. As mentioned in Chapter 3, government contributions and surplus funds from the Occupational Illness and Work Insurance Program are transferred into a Solidarity Fund which ICSS uses to subsidize health services in poor regions in Colombia. Contributions received from these regions are insufficient to cover the cost of providing health services. It would appear reasonable for the Government to fulfill its commitment to ICSS in this regard. Alternatively, employer and employee contributions may have to be raised. Since August 1972, a uniform schedule of rates has been in force throughout Colombia. The schedule formerly prevailing only in Antioquia, Valle, and Santa Marta, with minor adjustments, was applied to the rest of the country, where, rates had been somewhat lower.[13]

Conceptual and Statistical Limitations of the Analysis

While the willingness-to-pay approach deals with some of the conceptual limitations of the cost-of-service approach, some of the assumptions employed in the willingness-to-pay approach are also not beyond dispute.[14] The major conceptual issues relating to the cost-of-service approach concern: (1) the appropriate operational measure of redistribution and the general equilibrium problem, (2) the assumption that public services are optimally provided, (3) the identification of beneficiaries, (4) the evaluation of benefits, (5) limitation of the analysis to short run, impact measures of benefit incidence, and (6) endowment of the *status quo* with normative value. These issues were discussed in Chapter 2.[15]

Issues (1), (3) and (4) are dealt with in the willingness-to-pay analysis as follows: In most benefit incidence studies based upon the cost-of-service approach, the distribution of real income among households after government expenditures is compared with the distribution that would prevail in a no government economy. The general equilibrium problem is addressed in the willingness-to-pay approach by employing Musgrave's concept of "differential incidence" and by specifying which counterfactual appears to be the most appropriate. Redistribution is defined in this study as the difference between the Behrens and Smolensky *Lindahl II* primary distribution and the estimated final distribution of income.[16] In other words, the estimated distribution of after-tax factor income plus transfers and benefits of all final government services is compared with a primary distribution that arises from a Lindahl equilibrium, or the distribution that would prevail if benefit taxation were employed. In the willingness-to-pay approach, benefits are attributed not only to direct recipients, as in the cost-of-service approach, but also to indirect recipients. Finally, benefits are allocated across income classes on the basis of the utility received from public health programs rather than on the basis of the costs incurred on behalf of direct recipients.

Limitations of the cost-of-service approach listed, other than the three discussed above, also apply to the willingness-to-pay approach. First, total benefits are assumed to equal total costs, but this is only true if neither too little nor too much of the service is supplied and the public service is produced at constant average cost. A review of the evaluation procedure proposed by Aaron and McGuire will clarify the problem: They argue that the evaluation of publicly provided services should be placed upon an equal basis with the evaluation of private goods, which is based on relative prices.[17] Benefits from publicly provided health services need to be based upon marginal rates of substitution between these services and other goods and services or income. If decisions concerning public health expenditures have been *efficient*, or Pareto-optimal, then the marginal cost (MC) of the services equals the marginal benefit or, in the case of pure public goods, the sum of the marginal rates of substitution (MRS). Assuming that decisions have been Pareto-optimal, then total costs or the sum of the amounts that all households pay per unit of public good ($\Sigma\ t_i$) equals total benefits to be allocated to households ($\Sigma\ t_i = \Sigma$ MRS = MC), only if marginal and average costs are equal. If average costs are rising, benefits allocated will exceed budgetary costs; on the other hand, if average costs are falling, benefits allocated will fall short of budgetary costs. However, even if average costs are constant, budgetary costs will not equal total benefits allocated unless the service is provided at a Pareto-optimal level. If it is underprovided, marginal costs will exceed marginal benefits; conversely, if it is over-extended, marginal costs will fall below marginal benefits. Second, tax and benefit incidence studies estimate redistribution for a given year; however, even if tax and expenditure policies remain unchanged, the estimated effects may not be sustained over time due to general equilibrium effects. Furthermore, fiscal incidence studies are based upon the strong assumption that the utilities of individuals are derived from existing patterns of income, wealth, and talent, thus implicitly endowing the *status quo* with normative value.

In addition to the limitations discussed above, some issues may be raised concerning the willingness-to-pay approach itself.[18] This may apply to some of the following assumptions employed: (1) the treatment of source-of-income benefits, (2) the evaluation of in-kind transfers, and (3) the assumption that tastes are homogeneous throughout Colombia. Source-of-income benefits were added to use-of-income benefits in estimating total benefits for each income class. On the one hand, it may be argued that these are not additive. Whereas source-of-income benefits are analogous to factor payments, which constitute a means to utility rather than benefits themselves, use-of-income benefits are analogous to market values, indicating willingness and ability to pay for public health services. On the other hand, source-of-income benefits improve the welfare of recipients and may change the distribution of welfare across income classes. Adding source-of-income benefits to use-of-income benefits violates the accounting identity between costs and benefits, and this may be found to be disturbing by some.

In-kind transfers are assumed to generate benefits equal to their monetary value. This assumption is likely to overstate recipients' valuation of these benefits. However, no generally accepted procedure for determining the value placed upon them is currently available.

Finally, all utility functions may not be identical. If the utility of public goods declines with income, a smaller proportion of public goods benefits should be imputed to the well off. On the other hand, if the utility of public goods increases with private income, the reverse is true.

In addition to these conceptual difficulties, a number of technical problems were also confronted in distributing benefits and taxes by income class. For example, benefits generated by investment expenditures were assumed to equal costs incurred and allocated to the year in which they were made, although these may be expected to generate benefits in future years. It was assumed also that the access of different income classes to services rendered was equal.

Data on the distribution of personal income, consumption patterns, and socio-economic characteristics of users of health services provided in Colombia are far superior to those available in most other developing countries. However, the reliability of some of these data, is not knowable. For example, the income concept used in the household survey in theory includes both money income and income in kind, but whether, in fact, income in kind was taken into account is not known. Furthermore, the extent to which lower income households use the health services provided by ICSS and the Ministry of Public Health may be understated. The data for ICSS pertain only to individuals receiving subsidies due to incapacity to work. However, as mentioned earlier, this was the only method of obtaining income data for the recipients of health services without specifically requesting it from patients. In the case of the Ministry of Public

Health, only households which had paid for health services were considered recipients, whereas some very low income households may have received services without paying for them. However, charging for hospital services is a widespread practice, as mentioned earlier.

General Conclusion

Incidence studies can assist decision makers in formulating policies conducive to closing the gap between the existing and the desired income distribution in developing countries. Studies of the distributional implications of expenditures should be limited to partial incidence analysis of specific policy measures, as many now agree, rather than encompassing an analysis of the entire expenditure system, as was done in previous studies.[19] Most public policy decisions are concerned with marginal changes rather than an overhaul of the entire fiscal system. It is impossible to know the effect of an entire public finance system on the distribution of income, as it cannot be assumed that the existing distribution of income-before-tax would remain unchanged if the fiscal system did not exist. When smaller budget items are analyzed, this objection disappears, as marginal changes may be expected not to alter the distribution of income to such an extent as to make the results invalid.

Further research needs to be done into the willingness-to-pay approach, which is conceptually preferable to the standard method of measuring the benefits of public services. In particular, more research needs to be done on the evaluation of benefits from publicly provided services and on the decision-making process in specific countries. In studies of countries with effective mass participation in the political process, results estimated using the standard methodology may not diverge significantly from those obtained using the willingness-to-pay approach or they may be distributionally neutral. This would presumably also occur as incomes and preferences become less divergent.[20]

NOTES AND REFERENCES

[1] See Neenan, *Political Economy of Urban Areas*, pp. 102-03, for a summary of the Frey and Kohn analysis and Chapter 1, pp. 39-40.

[2] *Ibid.*, pp. 81-118.

[3] *Promotoras* are young women with a primary education who are provided short courses in simple health care, including first-aid,

injections, etc. and health education by the sectional health authorities. They are chosen by their communities and, after training, return to their communities to work.

[4] Instituto Nacional Para Programas Especiales de Salud, *Informe de Actividades: Agosto 1970-Julio 1974* (Bogota, D.E., Colombia: Instituto Nacional para Programas Especiales de Salud, 1975), p. 34.

[5] *Ibid.*, p. 36.

[6] USAID Mission to Colombia, "An Analysis of the Colombian Public Health Sector," pp. 165-179. (Xeroxed.)

[7] USAID Mission to Colombia, "1974 Colombian Health Sector Analysis" (Bogota, D.E., 1974), p. 204. (Xeroxed.)

[8] Legal authority to expand coverage to these groups was granted to ICSS with passage of the following Decree Law: Republica de Colombia, Ministerio del Trabajo, *Decreto Ley Numero 0433 de 1971*, 27 March 1971.

[9] Musgrave and Gillis, (eds.), *Fiscal Reform for Colombia: Final Report and Staff Papers of the Colombian Commission on Tax Reform.*

[10] In 1974, 712 million pesos were transferred under the *situado fiscal* for health: Contraloria General de la Republica de Colombia, *Informe Financiero de 1974* (Bogota, D.E., Colombia: Contraloria General de la Republica de Colombia, 1975), p. 178.

[11] Hans Schulten, "Patients, Physicians, and the Government," *Financing Medical Care: An Appraisal of Foreign Programs*, ed. Helmut Schoeck (Caldwell, Idaho: The Caxton Printers, Ltd., 1962), p. 166.

[12] Helmut Schoeck, "Introductory—Great Britain," *Ibid.*, p. 32.

[13] Republica de Colombia, Ministerio del Trabajo, *Decreto Numero 1036 de 1972*, 20 June 1972.

[14] The willingness-to-pay approach was developed by Greene, Neenan, and Scott, as mentioned earlier, and appears in: *Fiscal Interactions in a Metropolitan Area*, pp. 27-49.

[15] pp. 85-97.

[16] See Chapter 2, pp. 78-79.

[17] Aaron and McGuire, "Public Goods and Income Distribution," *op. cit.*, pp. 908-10.

[18] Greene, Neenan, and Scott, *Fiscal Interactions, op. cit.*, pp. 182-84.

[19] See Carl S. Shoup, *Public Finance* (Chicago: Aldine Publishing Company, 1970), p. 577; L. De Wulf, "Fiscal Incidence Studies," *op. cit.*, pp. 44-45.

[20] L. De Wulf, *Ibid.*, p. 48.

Appendix 1
THE THEORY OF EXPENDITURE INCIDENCE

Marginal differences in public and private expenditure patterns cause shifts in demand when resources are transferred from the private to the public sector and these demand shifts may be expected to cause changes in relative product and factor prices which will alter the distribution of income. As mentioned in Chapter 1, thorough examination of these effects requires the use of an adequately structured general equilibrium model. Theoretical partial or general equilibrium analysis of the incidence of government purchases of goods and services appears to be explicitly contained in the writings of only few economists. Among those who have undertaken theoretical analysis of expenditure incidence are: Antonio di Viti de Marco,[1] representing the Italian tradition in public finance, Richard A. Musgrave,[2] Osmo V. Jaskari,[3] and more recently, Charles E. McLure, Jr.[4] and Wayne R. Thirsk.[5] However, each of these economists, except McLure and Thirsk, was primarily concerned with the analysis of tax incidence. McLure constructed a comprehensive general equilibrium framework for analyzing expenditure incidence and employed it to examine how several expenditure programs affect the distribution of real incomes among individuals.[6] Since the model used was similar to the general equilibrium model of tax incidence developed by Harberger[7] and extended by Mieszkowski,[8] the analysis of expenditure incidence also was combined with an analysis of tax incidence. Subsequently, McLure and Thirsk employed the Harberger model to present in algebraic and numerical form an analysis of the distributional effect of shifts in expenditure patterns induced when purchasing power is transferred from the private to the public sector.[9]

The question of whether or not expenditure incidence analysis is needed at all in analyses of budgetary incidence and cost-benefit studies is disputed in the literature. Cost-benefit analyses typically disregard *pecuniary externalities*, as expenditure incidence (or changes in the distribution of income resulting from marginal differences in public and private spending patterns) is called, because these changes are entirely redistributional. In analyses of budgetary incidence, the appropriate treatment of expenditure incidence has produced contrasting opinions by important authorities on the subject. Musgrave has argued that governments should secure resources at least cost, and while these expenditures will help to determine relative factor and product prices, the resulting effects are unlikely to have a significant bearing on the size distribution of income in most cases.[10] Furthermore, he has argued that when public goods and services are purchased, how they will affect the distribution of earnings is not a major consideration. He therefore considers expenditure incidence less important than the incidence of tax and transfer policy. Musgrave recognizes, however, that government purchases may have important redistributional effects for particular industry groups, and that the redistributive effects of public expenditure may require special attention if redistribution cannot be carried out using other alternatives.[11]

In contrast to Musgrave, McLure asserts that expenditure incidence analysis is needed:[12]

(1) In order to maintain the desired distribution of income, even if all government expenditures were justified on the basis of efficiency. Musgrave's Distribution Branch would need to know how contemplated new expenditure programs or changes in existing programs would affect the distribution of income so that it could react to these changes.

(2) To determine whether public programs intended to redistribute income are, in fact, redistributing income in the desired way. McLure states that there is no reason to assume that government expenditures are efficient either from the point of view of using least cost production methods or from the point of view of having chosen the optimum mix and level of public goods. Many public programs are supported, however, despite costs due to inefficiency, because they are believed to redistribute income.

3) Because the redistributional effects of public expenditures may be important, particularly at the micro level and for different partitionings of income groups, e.g., by region. Pecuniary redistributions from public expenditures rather than just the benefits from public services, explain the existence of lobbies, influence peddling, and pork-barrel politics.

4) To determine the redistributional effects of such quasi-expenditure policies as conscription and confiscation. When governments conscript labor or transfer title to resources to the public sector through use of the power of eminent domain, land reform, or confiscation, compensation is not always at full market value.

Expenditure incidence occurs because the supply of that service to the private market has been reduced, thereby producing an effect comparable to increased market demand for the service by the government, while an implicit tax has been levied on the owners of the confiscated or conscripted service.

(5) In order to be able to select programs which might be marginally less efficient than alternative uses of resources but far more significant from a distributional point of view. Knowing how various public programs affect the distribution of income with regard to both expenditure and benefit incidence, we may provide services in a way that favors the poorest strata of the population.

As in the case of tax incidence analysis, three different approaches may be employed in expenditure incidence analysis: (1) *balanced budget* incidence, which involves the analysis of adjustments in both tax and expenditure policy in a balanced-budget context and the resulting effects on the distribution of income; (2) *differential* expenditure incidence, which involves a comparative analysis of the distributional effects of alternative public expenditure programs, assuming that tax functions remain unchanged; and (3) *specific* expenditure incidence, which is required when expenditures exceed taxes and therefore create inflation; it involves analysis of the distributional effects of both the expenditure and inflation.[13] In the case of the balanced-budget approach, the redistributive effects of an expenditure program of the government may be isolated by assuming that the program is financed by a general tax on all factors or on all products. Since the tax would reduce all incomes proportionately and therefore would not affect relative product or factor prices, any deviations from a sharing of the burden of the budget in proportion to the initial distribution of income could be attributed to differences in expenditure patterns of the private and the public sector.[14] In the case of specific expenditure incidence, the differential incidence of expenditures which are equally inflationary also could be analyzed.[15]

Theoretical analysis of expenditure incidence needs to take into consideration both the price effects and the employment effects of government expenditures. (See Figure 9.) In analyzing the effects of various government programs upon relative prices, and therefore upon the distribution of income, McLure employs the first and the third approaches listed above. His model consists of essentially the same basic assumptions and equations used in the general equilibrium model of tax incidence developed by Harberger and modified by Mieszkowski. He builds upon Musgrave's analysis of the effects of changes in budgeting policies upon the distribution of income which separates these into source-of-income effects and use-of-income effects.[16] (See Figure 10.) For example, individuals who spend a very large proportion of their incomes on goods whose prices have risen in relation to the prices of other goods lose on the use-of-income side. Loss on the source-of-income side may occur when individuals generate an exceptionally large proportion of their incomes by providing factor services the return to which has fallen relative to the return to other factor services. The determinants of these effects are discussed below,[17] and they are outlined in Figure 10.

When resources are transferred from the private to the public sector, the more disparate public and private spending patterns are at the margin, the greater are shifts in demand:

On the *use-of-income side*, demand shifts induce changes in relative prices of goods. The greater the shifts in demand, therefore, the greater the changes in relative prices and in the distribution of income. The change in the relative price of a given product is related inversely to both the elasticity of supply of the goods toward which demand has shifted and the price elasticity of demand for those goods. The greater the complementarity between the public and the private product in question, the greater the effect on the relative price of that product. These use-of-income effects on the distribution of income, *ceteris paribus*, will also be greater the more average consumer baskets among various households differ.[18]

On the *source-of-income* side, the production function and how it affects the elasticity of supply need to be examined in order to determine effects on relative factor rewards. The elasticity of supply is affected by factor mobility, intensities and substitutability.[19] The greater the factor mobility and the ease of substitution between factors, the more elastic is supply. If there is complete factor mobility, for example, in a two-factor two-good world, then the elasticity of supply varies with relative factor intensities in the two industries. In the cases of equal factor intensities and perfect substitution of factors in both industries, supply is perfectly elastic. In the cases of unequal factor intensities and imperfect substitution of factors, however, a budget-induced demand shift toward a labor-intensive product will benefit labor, while capital will lose. Given these changes in factor prices, the effect on the distribution of income then depends upon differences in the average composition of endowments of factor services in each group of households.[20]

Budget-induced shifts in demand may have particularly important redistributive effects if a factor, such as labor, is immobile. When demand is shifted to a particular region or industry, labour specific

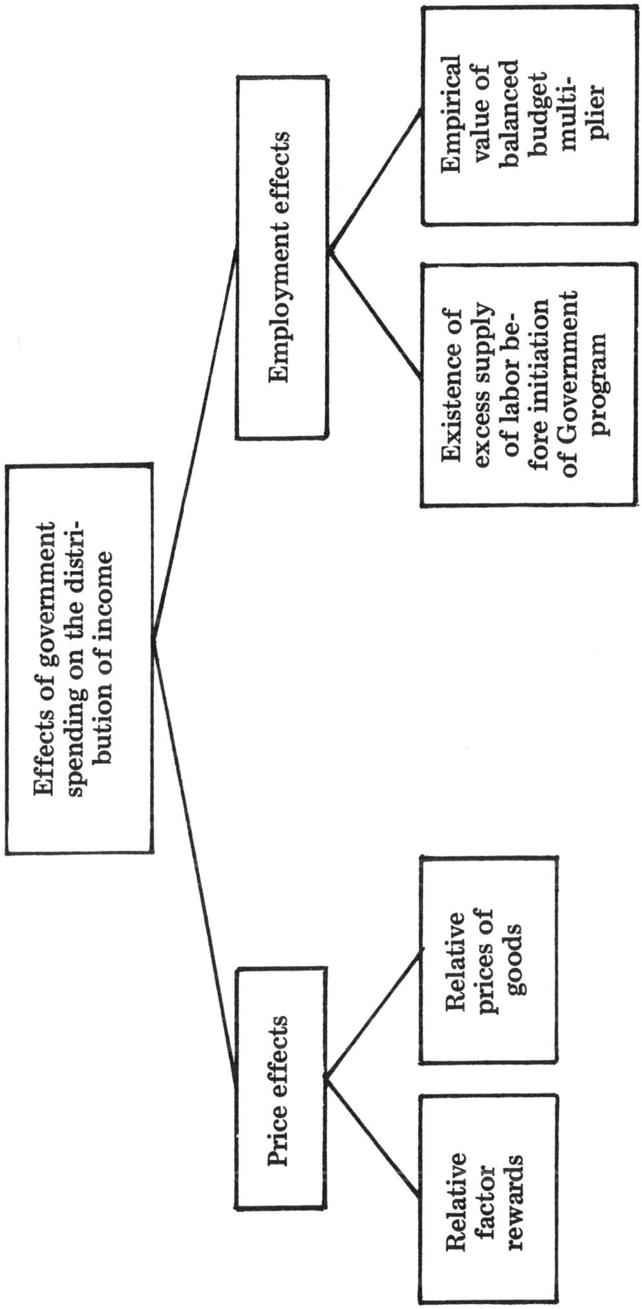

FIGURE 9: Expenditure incidence: price effects and employment effects.

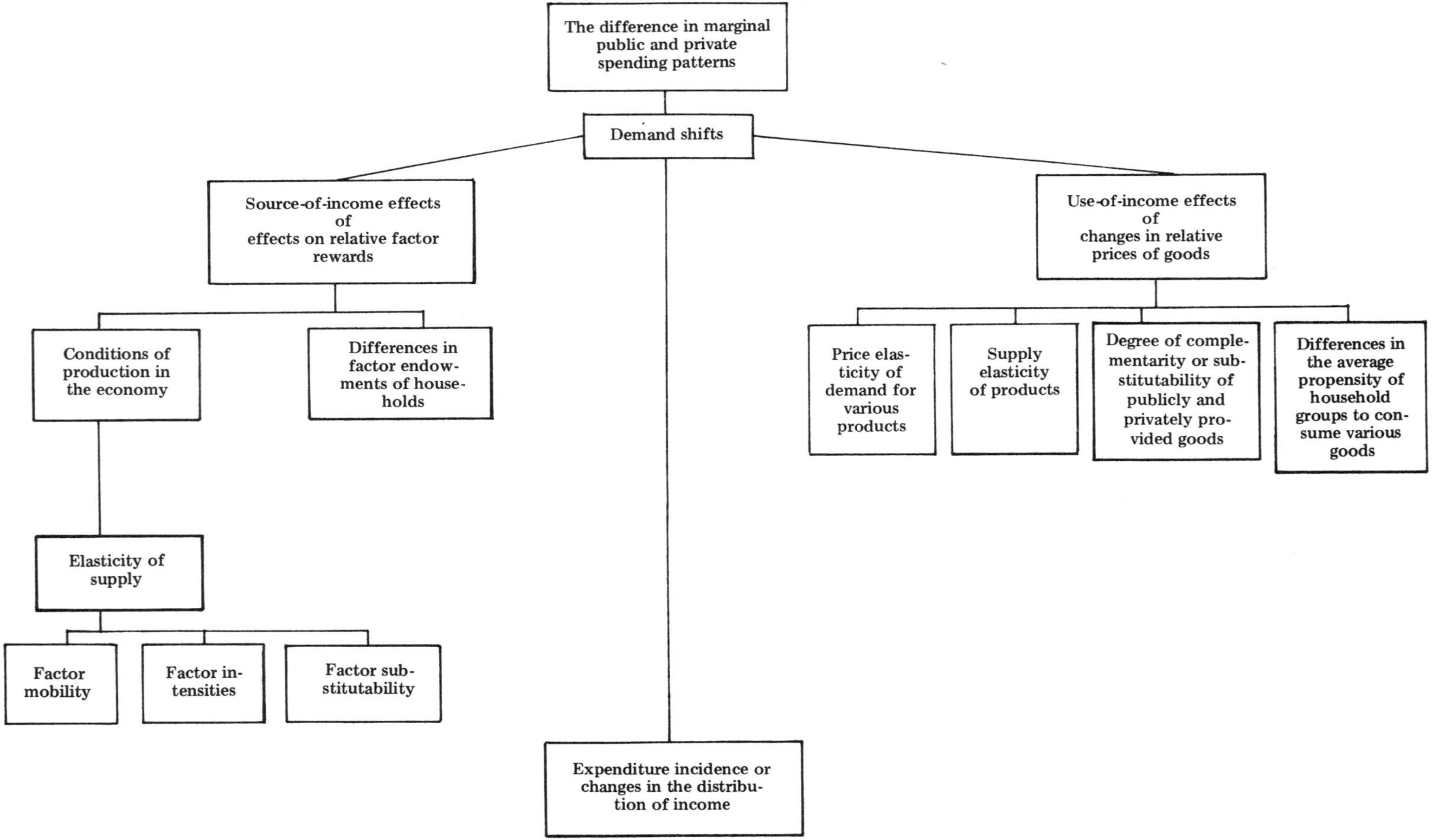

FIGURE 10: Expenditure incidence: determinants of the effects of government expenditures on relative prices.

to that industry or region may receive substantial rents and employment. Lobbyists clearly reveal the importance of factor immobility, at least in the short run, as they work to obtain government contracts for particular industries and regions. The size distribution of income may not be substantially affected by these effects, but the distribution of household income by regions, for example, may show important changes.[21]

The theoretical analysis of expenditure incidence has thus far focused upon price effects of expenditure incidence and assumed full employment, but the employment effects of public expenditures also need to be discussed. One of the primary goals of government spending in many instances is to reduce involuntary unemployment. The effect that government outlays may have on employment depends crucially upon the elasticity of supply of labor.[22] If supply is elastic, the employment effect may be substantial, but price effects are likely to be unimportant. On the other hand, if the supply of labor is inelastic, price effects and how these affect the distribution of income will be important, while the impact on unemployment will probably be small. If the employment effects of balanced budget operations are to be positive in the aggregate, that is, yield net benefits to society, there must not only be an excess supply of labor before the government program is initiated, but the balanced-budget multiplier must not be close to zero. Unless the impact upon aggregate employment is significant, however, the size distribution of income will probably not be substantially changed. But even if the impact upon aggregate employment is minor, the distributional effects for a different grouping of households, such as by regions, may be significant.

NOTES AND REFERENCES

[1] Summarized by James M. Buchanan, *Fiscal Theory and Political Economy* (Chapel Hill: University of North Carolina Press, 1960), pp. 24-74.

[2] Richard A. Musgrave, *The Theory of Public Finance* (New York: McGraw-Hill Book Co., 1959), pp. 213-14 and 355-57.

[3] Omo V. Jaskari, *A Study in the Theory of Incidence of Taxation* (Helsinki: Finnish Academy of Science, 1960).

[4] McLure, "The Theory of Expenditure Incidence," *op. cit.* pp. 432-53; and Charles E. McLure, Jr. and Wayne R. Thirsk with the assistance of Robert Klein, "A Simplified Exposition of the Harberger Model, II: Expenditure Incidence," *National Tax Journal* 28 (June 1975): 195-207.

[5] *Ibid.*

[6] McLure, "The Theory of Expenditure Incidence," *op. cit.*, pp. 437-47.

[7] Arnold C. Harberger, "The Incidence of the Corporation Income Tax," *Journal of Political Economy* 70 (June 1962): 215-40.

[8] Peter M. Mieszkowski, "On the Theory of Tax Incidence," *Journal of Political Economy* 75 (June 1967): 250-62.

[9] See McLure and Thirsk with the assistance of Klein, *op. cit.*, pp. 195-200; and a discussion of the analysis in: Benjamin Bridges, Jr., "The Harberger Incidence Model: A Comment," *National Tax Journal* 28 (December 1975): 462-66 and Charles E. McLure, Jr. and Wayne R. Thirsk, "The Harberger Model: Reply," *National Tax Journal* 28 (December 1975): 467-70.

[10] Musgrave, *The Theory of Public Finance*, *op. cit.*, p. 214; and Richard A. Musgrave and Peggy B. Musgrave, *Public Finance in Theory and Practice* (New York: McGraw-Hill, 1973), pp. 360-61.

[11] Musgrave and Musgrave, *ibid.*, pp. 156-59.

[12] McLure, "On the Theory and Methodology," *op. cit.*, pp. 36-38.

[13] Musgrave, *The Theory of Public Finance*, *op. cit.*, pp. 213-14.

[14] McLure, "The Theory of Expenditure Incidence," *op. cit.* p. 436.

[15] *Ibid.*

[16] Musgrave, *The Theory of Public Finance*, *op. cit.*, p. 217.

[17] This discussion summarizes McLure, "On the Theory and Methodology," *op. cit.*, pp. 39-42.

[18] *Ibid.*, p. 39.

[19] *Ibid.*, pp. 39-40.

[20] This point is discussed in Charles E. McLure, Jr., "Tax Incidence, Macroeconomic Policy and Absolute Prices," *Quarterly Journal of Economics* 84 (May 1970): 254-67.

[21] McLure, "On the Theory and Methodology," *op. cit.*, p. 40.

[22] *Ibid.*, pp. 41-43.

Appendix 2

THE LEVEL AND PATTERN OF PRIVATE EXPENDITURES ON HEALTH CARE, 1970

The 1970 survey of household expenditure patterns conducted by the Colombian statistical agency (DANE) provides the most complete information on private health care patterns of expenditures.[1] Table 32 summarizes the principal results of the health care survey for the seven large Colombian cities mentioned earlier in estimating the distribution of income in urban areas. The same procedure was used to blow up this information in order to make it representative of urban households in the entire country.

The level and pattern of expenditures on health services are strongly dependent on household income, as shown in the table.[2] While the highest 7 percent of the urban income distribution incurred expenditures of 4,810 pesos (U.S. $254) per year per household, the lowest 30 percent only spent 285 pesos (U.S. $15.05) per household per year.[3] Patterns of expenditure also appear to vary systematically with income. For example, drug purchases represent about half of all health expenditures in the lower income class but only about 22 percent in the highest income group. The converse is true for health insurance expenditures, which are relatively important for high-income households but constitute a relatively insignificant part of health expenditures for low-income households. Furthermore, the demand for health services also appears to be relatively elastic with respect to income at lower and middle income levels. The income elasticity for lower and middle income households appears to be about 1.27 but declines to about 0.92 for high income households.

Table 33 indicates the percentage of households in each income class that received the various types of health services listed. Demand for and/or access to health services appears to increase with income. Whereas only 2.6 percent of low-income households paid for dental services during the four-month survey period, 23.5 percent of high-income households paid for these services. The percentage of households paying for medical consultations is over 60 percent, on average,

Table 32: Private Health Expenditure Patterns in Urban Areas
By Income Class, 1970

	Household Income Class (Pesos/Year)				
	0-18,000	18,001-42,000	42,001-72,000	72,001-120,000	Over 120,000
Percent of total urban households	29.9	37.4	16.4	9.6	6.8
Average income (pesos)	11705	27241	52885	91169	188325
Average Health Expenditures	285	842	1694	2432	4810
Percent of Income spent on Health (%)	2.43	3.09	3.20	2.67	2.55
Composition of Health Expenditure (%):					
Drugs	49.6	39.5	33.0	25.8	21.8
Eyeglasses	0.7	1.0	2.2	1.4	0.8
Medical consultations	25.5	29.0	24.2	24.1	23.7
Medical treatment	1.7	3.6	3.2	4.9	6.5
Medical House calls	0.2	0.7	0.3	0.9	1.1
Dental Services	3.5	3.9	8.9	9.4	9.5
Ophthalmological services	-	0.3	0.2	0.7	0.4
Nursing services	1.3	0.6	1.4	1.0	1.5
Other medical services	0.1	0.5	0.6	0.6	0.1
Hospital clinical costs	2.6	5.8	7.4	9.5	10.6
Maternity costs	8.1	4.8	3.2	1.8	2.4
Pediatric costs	0.7	0.6	0.7	1.4	5.4
Laboratory tests	1.5	2.4	2.6	2.6	4.0
Ambulance services	0.1	0.1	-	-	-
Health & Accident Insurance	-	0.1	1.7	0.7	2.4
ICSS Contributions	3.4	4.2	4.7	3.9	2.9
Voluntary insurance	0.3	0.4	0.3	2.4	-
Government employees insurance	0.3	1.6	4.4	4.2	1.0
Other payments	0.2	1.0	0.8	4.9	5.9

Source: Departmento Administrativo Nacional de Estadistica (DANE), "Estructura del Consumo Relacionado Con la Salud," *boletin mensual de estadistica*, Nos. 264-265 (July-August, 1973), pp. 32-38.

TABLE 33: Households Purchasing Selected Health Services in Urban Areas
By Income Class, 1970

	0-18,000	18,001-42,000	41,001-72,000	72,001-120,000	Over 120,000
Number of Households (thousands)	610.0	764.3	334.5	195.9	137.9
Percent of Households purchasing:					
Drugs	52.7	67.5	66.3	70.7	68.3
Medical consultations	40.2	58.2	61.8	63.4	52.2
Dental services	2.6	8.0	13.3	19.3	23.5
Hospital clinical costs	1.9	3.4	3.5	5.4	23.5
Health insurance	4.4	13.0	23.9	26.4	15.7
From ICSS	3.9	9.2	14.5	14.2	8.6
Other	0.5	3.8	9.4	12.2	7.1

Source: Same as for Table 32.

for the three middle to upper income classes, as compared to only 40 percent for low-income families. If the survey results may be interpreted to imply that 60 percent of all households should have felt the need for at least one medical consultation during any four-month period, then it would appear that 20 percent of low-income households required medical consultation but did not have any. These figures probably understate the problem, however, as illness among low-income households tends to be more frequent than among middle and upper income groups.[4] Hospital-clinical costs also provide some interesting comparisons. About 2 percent of low-income households incurred hospital costs, 3 to 5 percent of middle and upper income groups, but about 24 percent of those in the highest income category. The use of health insurance also tends to rise with income. Households in the middle and upper-middle income ranges were the main purchasers of health insurance. In general, however, a relatively small proportion of households subscribe to health insurance programs in Colombia.

NOTES AND REFERENCES

[1] Departamento Administrativo Nacional de Estadistica (DANE), "Estructura del Consumo Relacionado Con la Salud," pp. 32-38.

[2] The results indicated in Table 32 are consistent with those obtained in: USAID Mission to Colombia, "An Analysis of the Colombian Public Health Sector," pp. 202-21, which attempted to expand the survey results to represent the country as a whole.

[3] The average exchange rate during the survey period was 18.93 pesos per U.S. dollar.

[4] USAID Mission to Colombia, "An Analysis of the Colombian Public Health Sector," *op. cit.*, p. 204.

SELECTED BIBLIOGRAPHY

Aaron, Henry, and McGuire, Martin. "Public Goods and Income Distribution." *Econometrica* 38 (November 1970): 907-20.

Andic, Fuat M. *Distribution of Family Incomes in Puerto Rico: A Case Study of the Impact of Economic Development on Income Distribution.* Puerto Rico: Institute of Caribbean Studies, University of Puerto Rico, 1964.

Arellano, Jose Pablo M. "El Gasto Publico en Salud y la Distribución del Ingreso." Estudios de Plantificación, Universidad Catolica de Chile, Documento No. 41, October 1974.

Behrens, Jean, and Smolensky, Eugene. "Alternative Definitions of Income Redistribution." *Public Finance* 28 (1973): 315-32.

Berry, Albert, and Padilla, Alfonso. "La Distribución de Ingresos Provenientes de la Agricultura en Colombia—1960." *boletin mensual de estadistica.* (DANE) (January 1971): xxi-xxvi.

Bhatia, Mohinder S. *Redistribution of Income Through the Fiscal System of Puerto Rico.* Puerto Rico: Puerto Rico Planning Board, 1960.

Bird, R.M., and DeWulf, L. "Taxation and Income Distribution in Latin America: A Critical Review of Empirical Studies." IMF *Staff Papers* 20 (November 1973): 639-82.

Boskoff, Alvin, and Zeigler, Harmon. *Voting Patterns in a Local Election.* Philadelphia: Lippincott, 1964.

Boulding, Kenneth E. "Notes on a Theory of Philanthropy." In *Philanthropy and Public Policy*, pp. 57-71. Edited by Frank G. Dickson. New York: National Bureau of Economic Research, 1962.

Bridges, Benjamin, Jr. "The Harberger Incidence Model: A Comment." *National Tax Journal* 28 (December 1975): 462-66.

Brittain, John A. "The Incidence of Social Security Payroll Taxes." *The American Economic Review* 61 (March 1971): 110-25.

________. "The Incidence of the Social Security Payroll Tax: Reply." *The American Economic Review* 62 (September 1972): 739-42.

________. *The Payroll Tax for Social Security.* Washington, D.C.: The Brookings Institution, 1972.

Bronfenbrenner, Martin. *Income Distribution Theory*. Chicago: Aldine—Atherton, Inc., 1971.

Buchanan, James M. *Fiscal Theory and Political Economy*. Chapel Hill: University of North Carolina Press, 1960.

_______. *Public Finance in Democratic Process: Fiscal Institutions and Individual Choice*. Chapel Hill: The University of North Carolina Press, 1967.

Buchanan, James M., and Tullock, Gordon. *The Calculus of Consent*. Ann Arbor: University of Michigan Press, 1965.

Burkhead, Jesse, and Miner, Jerry. *Public Expenditure*. Chicago: Aldine—Atherton, 1971.

Centro Estadistico Nacional de la Construccion. *El Poder Adquisitivo de los Salarios en Colombia: 1958-1974*. Bogotá, D.E.: Centro Estadistico Nacional de la Construccion, 1974.

Centro de Estudios sobre Desarrollo Economico. *Proyecciones de la Poblacion Colombiana: 1965-85*. Bogotá, D.E.: Centro de Estudios sobre Desarrollo Economico (CEDE), 1968.

Contraloria General de la Republica de Colombia. *Informe Financiero de 1970*. Bogotá, D.E.: Contraloria General de la Republica de Colombia, 1971.

_______. *Informe Financiero de 1974*. Bogotá D.E.: Contraloria General de la Republica de Colombia, 1975.

Córdova, Polibio. "Agregacion de Municipios a las Cuidades Investigadas en la Segunda Etapa de Encuesta de Hogares y Calculo de Factores de Expansión." Bogotá, D.E., 24 October 1972. (Xeroxed.)

_______. *Distribucion de Ingresos en Colombia*. Bogotá, D.E. "Departamento Administrativo Nacional de Estadistico (DANE), 1971.

________. *La Encuesta Nacional de Hogares de Colombia*. Bogotá, D.E.: Departamento Administrativo Nacional de Estadistica (DANE), 1971.

Departamento Administrativo Nacional de Estadistica (DANE). "Estructura del consumo relacionado con la salud." *boletin mensual de estadistica* 264-265 (July-August 1973): 32-38.

Devons, E. *Essays in Economics*. London: Allen & Unwin, 1961.

De Wulf, Luc. "Fiscal Incidence Studies in Developing Countries: Survey and Critique." IMF *Staff Papers* 22 (March 1975): 61-131.

Direccion General del Presupuesto. *Presupuesto de Colombia: 1970*. Bogotá, D.E.: Direccion General del Presupuesto, 1970.

Downs, Anthony. *An Economic Theory of Democracy*. New York: Harper & Row, 1957.

Dupuit, Jules. "On the Measurement of the Utility of Public Works." In *Readings in Welfare Economics*, pp. 255-83. Edited by Kenneth J. Arrow and Tibor Scitorsky. Translated by R. H. Barback. Homewood, Ill.: Irwin, 1969.

Estrada, Alcides. "Caracteristicas de las Mujeres que Solicitaron el Servicio de Planificacion Familiar en el Programa Materno Infantil de Ministerio de Salud Publica-Estadisticas de Servicio Primer Semestre de 1973." Paper prepared for the Ministerio de Salud Publica and the Centro Regional de Poblacion, Bogotá, D.E. December 1973. (Mimeographed.)

Feldstein, Martin S. "Net Social Benefit Calculation and the Public Investment Decision." *Oxford Economic Papers* 16 (March 1964): 114-31.

_______. "The Incidence of the Social Security Payroll Tax: Comment." *The American Economic Review* 62 (September 1972): 735-38.

_______. "Social Security, Induced Retirement, and Aggregate Capital Accumulation." *Journal of Political Economy* 82 (September/October 1974): 923-25.

Fellner, William. "Operational Utility: The Theoretical Background and a Measurement." In *Ten Studies in the Tradition of Irving Fisher*, pp. 39-74. New York: John Wiley and Sons, Inc., 1967.

Fisher, Irving. "A Statistical Method for Measuring 'Marginal Utility' and Testing the Justice of a Progressive Income Tax." In *Economic Essays, Contributed in Honor of John Bates Clark*. pp. 157-93. Edited by Jacob H. Hollander. New York: The Macmillan Co. Ltd., 1927.

Frey, Rene L., and Kohn, Leopold. "An Economic Interpretation of Voting Behaviour on Public Finance Issues." *Kyklos* 23 (1970) Fasc. 4: 792-805.

Friedman, Milton. "Transfer Payments and the Social Security System." *The Conference Room*. New York: Columbia University Press, 1965.

Frisch, Ragnar. "A Complete Scheme, for Computing All Direct and Cross Demand Elasticities in a Model with Many Sectors." *Econometrica* 27 (1959): 177-96.

Gillespie, W. Irwin. "Effect of Public Expenditures on the Distribution of Income: An Empirical Investigation." In *Essays in Fiscal Federalism*, pp. 122-86. Edited by Richard A. Musgrave. Washington, D.C.: The Brookings Institution, 1965.

________. *The Incidence of Taxes and Public Expenditures in the Canadian Economy*. Ottawa, Canada: Queen's Printer, 1966.

Goldfarb, R. S. "Pareto Optimal Redistribution: Comment. *The American Economic Review* 60 (December 1970): 994-96.

Greene, Kenneth V. "Collective Decision-Making Models and the Measurement of Benefits in Fiscal Incidence Studies." *National Tax Journal* 26 (June 1973): 177-85.

Greene, Kenneth V.; Neenan, William B.; and Scott, Claudia D. *Fiscal Interactions in a Metropolitan Area*. Lexington, Mass.: Lexington Books, 1974.

Groves, Harold M. *Financing Government*. 3d ed. New York: Henry Holt and Company, Inc., 1951.

Hansen, W. Lee, and Weisbrod, Burton A. "The Distribution of Costs and Benefits of Public Higher Education: The Case of California." *The Journal of Human Resources* 4 (Spring 1969): 176-91.

________. "Who Pays for a Public Expenditure Program?" *National Tax Journal* 24 (December 1971): 515-71.

Harberger, Arnold C. "The Incidence of the Corporation Income Tax." *Journal of Political Economy* 70 (June 1962): 215-40.

Hartman, Robert W. "A Comment on the Pechman-Hansen-Weisbrod Controversy." *The Journal of Human Resources* 5 (Fall 1970): 519-23.

Hochman, Harold M., and Rodgers, James D. "Pareto Optimal Redistribution." *The American Economic Review* 61 (1969): 542-57.

________. "Pareto Optimal Redistribution: Reply." *The American Economic Review* 60 (December 1970): 997-1002.

________. "Utility Interdependence and Income Transfers Through Charity." In *Transfers in an Urbanized Economy*, pp. 63-77. Edited by Kenneth E. Boulding, Martin Pfaff, and Anita Pfaff. Belmont: Wadsworth, 1973.

Instituto Colombiano de Seguros Sociales. *Cartilla del Seguro Social Obligatorio*. Bogotá, D.E.: Instituto Colombiano de Seguros Sociales, 1950.

________. *Estadistica de Casos de Incapacidad con Subsidios Pagados: Suplemento al Informe Estadistico: Año de 1971*. Bogotá, D.E.: Instituto Colombiano de Seguros Sociales, 1971.

________. *Informe del Director General: 1.970-1.971*. Bogotá, D.E.: Instituto Colombiano de Seguros Sociales, 1971.

________. *Informe Estadistico: 1971*. Bogotá, D.E. Instituto Colombiano de Seguros Sociales, 1972.

Instituto Nacional de Fomento Municipal. *Situacion Actual del Insfopal Dentro de las Instituciones del Sector Sanitario*. Bogotá, D.E.: Ministerio de Salud Publica, 1972.

Instituto Nacional Para Programas Especiales de Salud. *Informe de Actividades: Agosto 1970—Julio 1974*. Bogotá, D.E.: Instituto Nacional para Programas Especiales de Salud, 1975.

International Bank for Reconstruction and Development. *Economic Growth of Colombia: Problems and Prospects*. Baltimore: The Johns Hopkins University Press, 1972.

_______. *World Bank Atlas: Population, Per Capita Product and Growth Rates*. Washington, D.C.: International Bank for Reconstruction and Development, 1974.

Ireland, Thomas R. *The Economics of Charity*. Blacksburg: Center for the Study of Public Choice, 1970.

Jaskari, Omo V. *A Study in the Theory of Incidence of Taxation*. Helsinki: Finnish Academy of Science, 1960.

Jaszi, George. "A Critique of the United States Income and Product Accounts." In *Studies in Income and Wealth*, Vol. 22 pp. 13-127. Princeton: National Bureau of Economic Research, 1958.

Lindahl, Erik. "Just Taxation—a Positive Solution." (1919) In *Classics in the Theory of Public Finance*, pp. 168-76. Edited by Richard A. Musgrave and Alan T. Peacock. Translated by Elizabeth Henderson. London: Macmillan & Co. Ltd. 1962.

_______. "Some Controversial Questions in the Theory of Taxation." In *Classics in the Theory of Public Finance*, pp. 214-32. Edited by Richard A. Musgrave and Alan T. Peacock. Translated by Elizabeth Henderson. London: Macmillan & Co. Ltd., 1962.

McLure, Charles E., Jr. "On the Theory and Methodology of Estimating Benefit and Expenditure Incidence." Paper presented at the Workshop on "Income Distribution and Its Role in Development," William Marsh Rice University, Houston, Texas, 26 April 1974. (Xeroxed.)

_______. "Tax Incidence, Macroeconomic Policy and Absolute Prices." *Quarterly Journal of Economics* 84 (May 1970): 254-67.

_______. "The Incidence of Colombian Taxes, 1970." Paper No. 41, William Marsh Rice University, Houston, Texas, Summer 1973.

_______. "The Theory of Expenditure Incidence" *Finanzarchiv* 30 (1972): 432-53.

McLure, Charles E. Jr., Thirsk, Wayne R., ; with the assistance of Klein, Robert. "A Simplified Exposition of the Harberger Model, II: Expenditure Incidence." *National Tax Journal* 28 (June 1975): 195-207.

McLure, Charles E. Jr., and Thirsk, Wayne R. "The Harberger Model: Reply." *National Tax Journal* 28 (December 1975): 467-70.

McNamara, Robert S., President, World Bank Group. "Address to the Board of Governors." IBRD/IMF Annual Meeting, Washington, D.C. 25 September 1972. Washington, D.C.: International Bank for Reconstruction and Development, 1972.

Maital, Shlomo. "Is Redistributive Taxation a Myth?" Discussion Paper No. 122, Institute of Economic Research, Queens University, Kingston, Ontario, January 1973.

———. "Public Goods and Income Distribution: Some Further Results." *Econometrica* 41 (May 1973): 561-68.

Manrique, Rodrigo. "The Incidence of Public Expenditures in Colombia." Master's thesis, Vanderbilt University, 1972. (Xeroxed.)

Marglin, Stephan A. "The Social Rate of Discount and the Optimal Rate of Investment." *Quarterly Journal of Economics* 77 (1963): 95-111.

Mazzola, Ugo. "The Formation of the Prices of Public Goods." (1890) In *Classics in the Theory of Public Finance*, pp. 37-47. Edited by Richard A. Musgrave and Alan T. Peacock. Translated by Elizabeth Henderson. London: Macmillan & Co. Ltd., 1962.

Mera, K. "Experimental Determination of Relative Marginal Utilities." *Quarterly Journal of Economics* 83 (August 1969): 464-77.

Meyer, P. A., and Shipley, J. J. "Pareto Optimal Redistribution: Comment." *The American Economic Review* 60 (December 1970): 988-90.

Mieszkowski, Peter M. "On the Theory of Tax Incidence." *Journal of Political Economy* 75 (June 1967): 250-62.

Ministerio de Hacienda y Credito Publico. Dreccion General del Presupuesto, Division de Estudios Presupuestales, *Boletin de la Direccion General del Presupuesto: No. 62—Diciembre de 1972.* Bogotá, D.E.: Imprenta Nacional, 1973.

Ministerio de Salud Publica and Associación de Facultades de Medicina. *Investigación Nacional de Morbilidad: Atencion Medica.* Bogotá, D.E.: Asociacion de Facultades de Medicina and Ministerio de Salud Publica, 1968.

Ministerio de Salud Publica. *informe al honorable congreso de la republica de Colombia: 1972-1973.* Bogotá, D.E.: Ministerio de Salud Publica, 1974.

Mishan, E. J. "Evaluation of Life and Limb: A Theoretical Approach." *Journal of Political Economy* 79 (July/August 1971): 687-705.

———. "The Futility of Pareto-Efficient Distributions." *The American Economic Review* 62 (December 1972): 971-76.

Musgrave, R.A. "Pareto Optimal Redistribution: Comment." *The American Economic Review* 60 (December 1970): 991-93.

_______. "Provision of Social Goods." In *Public Economics*, pp. 124-44. Edited by J. Margolis and H. Guitton. London: Macmillan & Co. Ltd., 1969.

_______. *The Theory of Public Finance*. New York: McGraw-Hill Book Co., 1959.

Musgrave, R. A.; Carroll, J. J.; Cook, L.D.; and Frane, L. "Distribution of Tax Payments by Income Groups: A Case Study for 1948." *National Tax Journal* 4 (March 1951): 1-53.

Musgrave, Richard A., and Gillis, Malcolm, eds. *Fiscal Reform for Colombia: Final Report and Staff Papers of the Colombian Commission on Tax Reform.* Cambridge, Mass.: Harvard Law School International Tax Program, 1971.

Musgrave, Richard A. and Musgrave, Peggy. *Public Finance in Theory and Practice*. New York: McGraw-Hill, 1973.

Mushkin, Selma J. "Health as an Investment." *Journal of Political Economy* 70 (October 1962): 129-57.

Neenan, William B. "Income Redistribution through Local Government Fiscs." Discussion Paper No. 290-75, Institute for Research on Poverty, University of Wisconsin, Madison, Wisconsin, July 1975.

_______. *Political Economy of Urban Areas.* Chicago: Markham Publishing Company, 1972.

Parra, Horacio Escobar, "Programa Coordinado de Extension de la Seguridad Social al Sector Campesino." *Seguridad Social* 20 (September-December 1971): 277-312.

Pechman, Joseph A. "The Distributional Effects of Public Higher Education in California." *The Journal of Human Resources* 5 (Summer 1970) 361-70.

Pigou, A.C. *A Study in Public Finance*. Rev. 3d ed. London: Macmillan and Co. Ltd., 1962.

Piven, Frances Fox, and Cloward, Richard A. *Regulating the Poor.* New York: Pantheon Books, 1971.

Powell, Alan A.; Van Hoa, Tran.; and Wilson, R. H. "A Multi-Sectoral Analysis of Consumer Demand in the Post-War Period." *The Southern Economic Journal* 35 (October 1968): 109-20.

Republica de Colombia, Gobierno Nacional. *Ley 90 de 1946*. 26 December 1946.

Republica de Colombia, Ministerio del Trabajo. *Decreto Numero 2690 de 1960*. 23 November 1960.

_______. *Decreto Numero 3170 de 1964* 21 December 1964.

_______. *Decreto Numero 3041 de 1966.* 19 December 1966.

———. *Decreto Ley Numero 0433 de 1971.* 27 March 1971.

———. *Decreto Numero 1036 de 1972.* 20 June 1972.

Ridker, R. G. *The Economic Costs of Air Pollution.* New York: Praeger, 1967.

Samuelson, Paul A. "Pure Theory of Public Expenditure and Taxation." In *Public Economics*, pp. 98-123. Edited by J. Margolis and H. Guitton. London: Macmillan & Co. Ltd., 1969.

Sato, Kazuo. "Additive Utility Functions with Double-Log Consumer Demand Functions." *Journal of Political Economy* 80 (January/February): 102-24.

Schelling, T. C. "The Life You Save May be Your Own." In *Problems in Public Expenditure Analysis*, pp. 127-62. Edited by Samuel B. Chase, Jr. Washington, D.C.: The Brookings Institution, 1968.

Schmundt, M.; Smolensky, E., and Stiefel, L. *The Evaluation by Recipients of In-Kind Transfers.* Madison: University of Wisconsin, Institute for Research on Poverty, 1974.

Schoeck, Helmut. "Introductory-Great Britain." In *Financing Medical Care: An Appraisal of Foreign Programs*, pp. 29-34. Edited by Helmut Schoeck. Caldwell Idaho: The Caxton Printers, Ltd., 1962.

Schulten, Hans. "Patients, Physicians, and the Government." In *Financing Medical Care: An Appraisal of Foreign Programs*, pp. 151-71. Edited by Helmut Schoeck. Caldwell, Idaho: The Caxton Printers, Ltd., 1962.

Shoup, Carl S. *Public Finance*, Chicago: Aldine Publishing Company, 1970.

Snodgrass, Donald R. "The Fiscal System as an Income Redistributor in West Malaysia." Economic Development Report No. 224, Development Research Group, Harvard University, Cambridge, 1972.

Tanzi, Vito. "Fiscal Reform for Colombia: The Report of the Musgrave Commission." *Inter-American Economic Affairs* 26 (Summer 1972): 71-80.

The Urban Institute. "Unscrambling Metropolitan Fiscal Flows" *Search: A Report from the Urban Institute* 4 (January-April 1974): 3-8.

Urrutia, Miguel. "La Distribucion de Ingresos en Colombia." Bogotá, D.E.: Banco de la Republica. (Xeroxed).

Urrutia, Miguel M., and de Sandoval, Clara E. "Politica Fiscal y Distribucion del Ingreso en Colombia." *Revista del Banco de la Republica.* (Bogotá) 44 (July 1971): 1072-87.

USAID Mission to Colombia. "An Analysis of the Colombian Pubiic Health Sector." Bogotá, D.E., December 1972.

_______. "1974 Colombian Health Sector Analysis." Bogotá, D.E., 1974. (Xeroxed).

Vickrey, William S. "One Economist's View of Philanthropy." In *Philanthropy and Public Policy*, pp. 31-56. Edited by Frank G. Dickinson. New York: National Bureau of Economic Research, 1962.

Watson, Richard A. *The Politics of Urban Change*. Kansas City: Community Studies, Inc., 1963.

Watts, William, and Free, Lloyd A. *State of the Nation*. New York: Universe Books, 1973.

Wilson, James Q., and Banfield, Edward C. "Voting Behaviour on Municipal Public Expenditures: A Study in Rationality and Self-Interest." In *The Public Economy of Urban Communities*, pp. 74-91. Washington D.C.: Resources for the Future, 1975.

World Bank. *Health: Sector Policy Paper.* Washington, D.C.: World Bank, 1975.

INDEX

Aaron, H. and McGuire, M.: 41; benefits from public goods to income classes, 49; imputation of benefits, 40, 41, 83, 137; measurement of benefits from public goods, 28; selection of utility function, 34-37; willingness-to-pay principle, 40, 49

Aaron and McGuire Theorem: 137; 167; defined, 28; exposition of, by Maital, 28-34; illustrated, 188

Allocation of benefits to income classes: limitation of cost-of-service method, 77-86, 187; limitations of willingness-to-pay method, 87, 188-189

Allocation of resources: based on distribution of benefits, 15

Andic, F.: benefits in fiscal incidence studies, 65; incidence of public health expenditures, Puerto Rico, 1955, 71-72; public health expenditures, Puerto Rico, 1955; 71, 72

Antioquia: 187, sectional office of, 151

Arellano, J.: fiscal incidence study, 65; incidence of public health expenditures, Chile, 1969, 75

Argentina: distribution of income, 124

ASCOFAME. *See* Colombian Association of Medical Faculties

Australia: measure of elasticity of substitution among goods, 35

Balanced budget multiplier, 199

Balanced budget incidence: 21; in expenditure incidence analysis, 195

Basel-Stadt, Switzerland: 40; public finance referenda in, 39, 55, 180; willingness-to-pay principle in, 38

Behrens, J. and Smolensky, E.: 78-82; counterfactual preference, 82; definition of Lindahl II, 80; evaluation of Lindahl I vs. Lindahl II variations, 81; income redistribution studies, 78; Lindahl counterfactual defined, 91; Lindahl equilibrium, 79; Lindahl II counterfactual, 87; Lindahl II primary distribution, 187; reaction to Smolensky-Behrens counterfactual, 81; variants of Lindahl distribution, proposed, 79

Beneficiaries: identification of as limitation in cost-of-service method, 77, 83

Benefit incidence analysis: 179; 180; defined, 17; development of theory of, 48; investment expenditure, 46, 47, 48; limitation of analysis of short-run impact measures, 187; pattern of, 181; use in developing countries, 190

Benefit principle: deviations from, as cause for redistribution of Lindahl I, 79

Benefit theory of taxation, 28

Benefit weight: defined, 21

Benefits: evaluation of, 187-188

Benefits generated by governmental expenditures: 20; cost-of-service approach, 66-67; identification of, 87; individual basis of, 18, 51; private, 23-24; public nonredistributive, 23-24; public redistributive, 23-24-27; source-of-income, 19, 21-22; use-of-income, 22-48; willingness-to-pay approach, 37-40

Berry, A. and Padilla, A.: distribution of agricultural income, 174

Bhatia, M.: 73; benefit approach to allocating benefits, 66; effective benefit ratio, Puerto Rico, 72-73; fiscal incidence study, 65; incidence of public health expenditures, Puerto Rico, 1958, 72; money flow approach, 66

Board of Administration: established for rural sanitation projects, 101

Boards of Directors, Colombian health agencies, 96

Bogotá, Hospital San Juan de Dios, 74

Bogotá, Special District of, 185

Boskoff, A. and Zeigler, H.: willingness-to-pay principle, 38

Boyaca, 110

British government: financing of National Health Service, 186

Brittain, J.: bearers of social security tax, 149; Feldstein's response to

study of, 150; impact of employers tax on wage rates, 149; incidence of employer tax, social security contributions, 146; response to Feldstein's criticism, 150-151
Buchanan, J.: fiscal residual, 176
Budget incidence analysis, 193

Cajas de Prevision Social, 94
Canada: fiscal incidence studies, 65; Gillespie study, 67; measure of elasticity of substitution among goods, 35; sanitation expenditures, 69; study of public expenditures for hospital care, 68
Canadian Hospital Insurance Plan, 68
Central government of Colombia allocation of revenue, 185; subsidization services for poor, 172-173; tax collections of 169-170
Ceteris paribus, 196
Chile, 82; distribution of income in, 124; fiscal incidence studies, 65; incidence of public health expenditures, Arellano, 75
Clark, J.: economic value of human life, 57
Coffee export duties: allocation of, 170; bearers of, 124; McLure assumptions in analysis of, 175
Coffee exports: taxes on, 130
Coffee tax: allocation of by income group, 130; effect on household income, 130
Colombia: analysis of distribution of public health benefits, 119; analysis of redistributive impact, 119; bearers of corporate income tax, 180; bearers of social security tax, 151; benefit incidence of public health expenditures, 118; causes of morbidity and mortality in, 95; ceding of income to spouse, 126; changes in tax system, 184; citizen attitudes toward public health programs, 180; consumers and corporate income tax, 129; consumers, as bearers of corporate income tax, 170; development goals, 92-93; development strategy, 114; distribution of household income in urban areas, 119, 120; distribution of income, 118, 119; distribution of income among households, 120, 170; distribution of income compared with other Latin American countires, 124; employment policies, 92; expansion of Colombian Social Security Institute services, 110; fiscal incidence study, 65; future of health policy in, 179; health policies and institutions in, 114, 181; improvement of income distribution, 93; incidence of national taxes, 119, 132; incidence of public health expenditures in, 16; leading causes of death in, 97; malaria in, 102; management of INPES program, 182; marginal evaluation of public health services, 84; maternal child care program, 96, 114, 135, 139, 140, 141, 171, 172, 181, 182; poor regions in, 187; president's selections to Board of Directors, Colombian Social Security Institute (ICSS), 109; price discrimination for hospital services, 185; progressivity of tax system, 132; public health expenditure in. *See* Public health expenditures; public health policy makers, 92; public health sector in, 17; public service provision, urban areas, 101; redistributional impact of public health expenditures in, 179; regions covered by ICSS, 115; reliability of data for study of, 189; sanitation in, 100; shareholders in, 124; shareholders in, as bearers of corporate income tax, 170; strategy for growth in cities of, 102; subscribers to health insurance in, 204; tastes in, as assumptions in willingness-to-pay approach, 188-189; tax incidence, 16; total income distribution for nation, 120; transmittable diseases in, 100; upper income shareholders, 129; vaccination campaigns in, 100, 102
Colombian Agrarian Reform Institute (INCORA): funder for coordinated rural health programs, 112; implementors of medical-social survey, 112; lender to landowners, 112; sponsor of health services to self-employed rural workers, 110
Colombian Association of Medical Faculties (ASCOFAME): national health survey conducted, 1965-1966, 95
Colombian Commission on Tax Reform (Musgrove Commission), 184
Colombian Family Welfare Institute (ICBF): establishment of, 97
Colombian health programs: distribution of income, 16
Colombian-made goods, 93
Colombian Social Security Institute

(ICSS): 93; 94; 113; 118; 159; 180; analysis of incidence of health expenditures, 169; analysis of medical care provided by, 184; beneficiaries of health services, 172; benefits allocated by income class, 173; Board of Directors for, 109; distribution of income among employees covered by 144; employee contributions to, 151; employer contributions to, 151; expenditures of, 17, financial resources of, 114, 144, 154, 172, 186, financing of National Hospital Fund, 112; function of, 104, 114, 141, 144; funding for coordinated rural health program, 112; health services provided by, 114; incidence of benefits generated by health expenditures, 157; 167; incidence of employer tax, 146; limited coverage of agricultural workers, 146; percentage of total Colombian health expenditure, 115; physicians employed by, 154; private sector employees affiliated with, 154; programs of, 105; programs in Quindio, 1950, 110; provision of use-of-income benefits, 167; redistributional impact of Colombian health expenditure, 179; regions covered by, 115; revenues of, 104; sale of bonds to, 95; socio-economic information on beneficiaries of health services provided by, 154, 157, 159; statistics compiled by, 157; system of disease classification, 157; taxes levied by, 180; use-of-services provided by, 189; utilization of Solidarity Fund, 187

Colombian Statistical Agency (DANE): data on income distribution among rural population, 120; household consumption survey, 130, 170, 171, 201; possible survey errors, 124; seven cities survey, 151; survey of income distribution, 119, 170; survey results, 124

Colombian ten-year health plan, (PAHO), 95

Comisarias, 185

Community Action group: 93; rural sanitation project, 101

Compensating variation: in evaluating loss or saving of life, 60

Constant elasticity of substitution (CES), 149

Coordinated Rural Health Program, 110

Corporate income tax: allocation of, 170; assumption used in allocation to income class, 129; bearer of 129, 132, 171, 180; incidence of, 129; non-Colombian shareholders, 129

Cost benefit studies, 193

Cost equal benefits: as limitation of cost-of-service method, 86

Cost-of-service: 181-182; as basis for fiscal residual calculations, 141; benefits, estimates of, 169; distribution of benefits generated by public health services, 76; estimates, 140, 172, 180, 184; incidence of benefits based on, 172; methodology, limitations of, 77

Cost-of-service approach: conceptual limitations of, 187-188

Cost-of-service basis: analysis of distribution of benefits, 144; benefit incidence estimated on, 118; benefits estimated on, 157; benefits from health services estimated on, 135; estimation of distributions of benefits from health services, 157

Cost-of-service method: 87; benefits imputed from, 83; expenditures allocated to income groups using, 157; identification of beneficiaries, 83; in allocation of benefits generated by health expenditures, 132; results of benefit incidence under, 181; shortcomings of, 86; used in health expenditure analysis, 171; used to allocate benefits, 179; used to determine ICSS benefits by income class, 173

Cost of services: Greene, Neenan & Scott, 66

Counterfactual: choice of, as limitation of cost-of-service method, 77

Cundinamarca: sectional office of, 151

Current expenditures: combined with investment expenditures, 135

Customs duties: 130; allocation of, 171

Customs duties and stamp taxes: allocation of, 131

DANE. *See* Colombian Statistical Agency

Data: limitations of, 179

Death benefits: introduction of, 144

Decree 477, 100

Decree 1423, 95

Decree 1499, 96

Decree 2470, 96

Decree 3178, 102
Decree 3224: health attention concept, 94-95
DeKalb County, Georgia: voter survey, 54
Demand shifts: redistributive effects of, 196
De Marco, A.: theoretical analysis of of expenditure incidence, 193
Department of Huila, 113
Department of Meta, 112
Departmental governor: head of sectional health service, 115
Development expenditures, 74
De Wulf, L.: characteristics of beneficiaries, 157
Differential expenditure incidence: 21; in tax incidence analysis, 195
Direct cost sharing of medical care, 186
Direct tax: allocation of, 170; defined, 126
Distribution of income: governments' role in, 15
Dupuit, J.: willingness-to-pay principle, 37, 85

Economic value of human life: measured, 57
Ecuador: distribution of income in, 124
Education: governmental expenditure on, 56
Effective tax rates: estimated, 171
Elasticity of substitution among goods for eight nations, 35
Engel, E.: economic value of human life, 57
Enterprises for Potable Water for Santiago and El Canelo, Chile, 75
Epidemic disease: national campaign against, 183
Epidemiology: as expenditure of Ministry of Health, 171; expenditures on, 135
Exhaustive expenditures: analysis of, 19-22, 79; as government expenditure, 19
Expenditure incidence: defined, 17; effect of government expenditure on, 195; employment effects of, 199; use for analysis of, 193-195

Factor payments: analogous to source-of-income benefits, 189; effect on net income, 48-49; net income gains from, 21
Farr, W.: economic value of human life, 57
Feldstein, M.: 46-48; and social security, 177; criticism of Brittain's study, 150; net addition to consumption, 50
Fellner, W.: 35; 38; 40; analysis of, 139; estimation of elasticity of marginal utility, 36; willingness-to-pay principle, 49-50
Final distribution: Behrens and Smolensky, 78
Fiscal incidence: 179; defined, 17
Fiscal residuals: and attitude toward government expenditures, 38-40; Buchanan, 176; calculation of, 141; defined, 26; defined by Neenan, 39; derivation of, 180; determinant of willingness-to-pay, 39; estimation on cost-of-service basis, 169, 180; estimation on willingness-to-pay basis, 169, 180; function of, 141; per worker, 169
Fisher, I.: 36; economic value of human life, 57; study of tax incidence and equity, 34
Frey, R. and Kohn, L.: analysis of public finance referenda, 39, 180-181
Friedman, M.: incidence of employer tax, 146
Frisch, R.: measurement of income elasticity of marginal utility, 34

Gasoline tax: 130; allocation of, 170; attributed to, 131; petroleum subsidy, 175
GDP: 16; in estimate of income distribution, 74-75; total government expenditures of, 87
General equilibrium adjustment: 19; initiated by government, 21
General equilibrium model, 193
General equilibrium problem, 187
General Health and Maternity Insurance, 104; contributions to, 151; ICSS contributions to, 144; ICSS provisions under, 114; subsidies paid, 110
General sales tax, 130
Germany: health insurance in, 185; reformation of health service, 186
Gillespie, W.: 68; 73; 78-79; 83; 151; beneficiaries of Canadian sanitation expenditures, 69; Canadian hospital care expenditures, 69; Canadian public health expenditures, 68; estimates of net incidence of U.S. taxes and expenditures, 1960, 25; estimates of waste, 88; fiscal incidence studies, 65; income

concepts, illustrated, 71; results of incidence of public health and sanitation expenditure, 71; study of tax and public expenditure incidence, 67; zero budget counterfactual, 78
Gini coefficient, 124
Government action, 93
Government activity: revenues and expenditure aspects of, 17
Government budgetary policies: impact on distribution of income, 15
Government expenditures: benefits allocated by income class, 16; distributional impact of, 16; effect on individual welfare, 18-19, 48; evaluation of benefits of, 18; exhaustive expenditures, 19; money transfer, 19; source-of-income benefits, 19; use-of-income benefits, 22
Government services: benefits of, 78
Greene, K., Neenan, W. and Scott, C.: application of Maital's formula, 137; assumption for total expenditures, 80-81; cost-of-services, 66; criticism of Hochman and Rodgers paper, 27; current expenditures, 82; decision making process, 44; estimation of nontransfer and donor benefits, 81; first component of distribution, 81; fiscal incidence study, 65; individual utility, 85; level of public services, 88; Lindahl II, 80-81; Lindahl II counterfactual, 87; Maital's general function form, 137; marginal benefits vs. marginal cost of collective service, 41; pattern of benefit incidence, 77; public health expenditures, Washington, D.C., 76; recipient benefits of Pareto transfers, 81; utility function, 34; willingness-to-pay principle, 37-40, 50, 77, 83, 86
Gross National Product: increase in, 15
Gross output: in evaluating loss or saving of life, 58-59
Groves, H.: incidence of employer tax, 146

Harberger, A.: general equilibrium model, 193
Health expenditures: 74; financing of, 179; incidence of benefits generated by, 132
Health insurance expenditures: pattern of, 201; purchasers by income class, 204
Health Post and Health Centers: staffing of, 113
Health sector: capital stock in, 135
Health service expenditure pattern, 201
Health services: analysis of distribution of benefits generated by, 137, 140-141, 157, 167; demand for access to, 201; financing of, 94; objectives of, 109
Health systems: regionalization of, 183
Hochman, H. and Rodgers, J.: Pareto criterion analysis, 25-26; reply to Musgrave criticism, 27; paper, 26
Hospital admissions, leading causes of, 97
Hospital centers: determination of patients to be admitted to, 113
Hospital facilities, location of, 73
Hospital San Juan de Dios: patients' income class distribution at, 74

ICBF. *See* Colombian Family Welfare Institute
ICSS. *See* Colombian Social Security Institute
Illness: economic cost of, 92; tendency for as related to income class, 159
Incapacity: causes of, 159, 167
Income concept: defined, 119
Income of poor: raising of, 15
INCORA. *See* Colombian Agrarian Reform Institute
Indirect tax: 130; allocation of by income class, 170
Individualistic approach: defined, 18, 51
In-kind transfers: 19; 21; 24; 118; as cause for redistribution of Lindahl I, 79; as source-of-income benefit, 48; distinct from "spillover" benefits, 23; for beneficiaries of Washington, D.C. public health expenditures, 76; forms of, 21; source-of-income benefits from, 139; generation of benefits, 189; in willingness-to-pay principle, 188; measurement of welfare gain, 21; recipient benefits, 78
INPES. *See* National Institute of Special Health Programs
INSFOPAL. *See* National Institute for Municipal Development
Insurance principle: defined, 59; in evaluating loss or saving of life, 59
Intendencias, 185
Invalidism benefits, 144
Investment expenditures: benefit incidence of, 46; benefits generated

by, 82, 189; use-of-income benefits from, 50
Israel: measure of elasticity of substitution among goods, 35

Japan: measure of elasticity of substitution among goods, 35
Jaskari, O.: theoretical analysis of expenditure incidence, 193
Jaszi, G.: incidence of employer tax, 146

Kansas City, Missouri: willingness to pay in, 55
Kantian motive: willingness-to-pay principle, 24

Latin America: vaccination campaigns in, 100
Law 90, 1946, 104
Lindahl, E.: benefit theory of taxation, 28-29
Lindahl distribution: defined, 79
Lindahl equilibrium: defined, 79; primary distribution from, 187
Lindahl I counterfactual: efficient transfers in, 80; defined, 79; limitations of, 79; preferred by Behrens and Smolensky, 82; redistribution relative to, 79, 91; vs. zero-budget counterfactual, 79
Lindahl II counterfactual: defined, 80; McLure's preference for, 82
Lorenz curve, 123-124; for income distribution in urban and rural areas, 120
Luxury items: taxing of, 132

McLure, C.: adjustments to DANE survey, 119, 124; analysis of government program on distribution of income, 195, 196; benefit ratios in Colombia, 74; characteristics of beneficiaries, 157; counterfactual preference, 82; evaluation of Smolensky-Behrens counterfactual, 81; expenditure incidence analysis, 194-195; general equilibrium model, 21; income distribution, 73; income distribution pattern, 120; limitation of Lindahl I, 80; Lindahl I, response to, 80; possible error in DANE survey, 124; theoretical analysis of expenditure incidence, 193; zero government world, 79
McNamara, R.: study of benefit incidence, 16
Maital, S.: 37-40; form for marginal utility of income, 83-84, 167; general functional form, 137; income elasticity of marginal utility for United States, 34-35, 36-37; willingness-to-pay principle, 49
Malaria: Colombian climate conducive to, 102
Manrique, R.: 83; beneficiaries by income group, 73; estimation of benefit ratios, 74; fiscal incidence studies, 65; public health expenditures, 73
Marginal utility: elasticity of, 167, 172, 176, 178; income elasticity of, 76, 139; measurement of relation to income, 28-29
Maternal/child care: 114; as expenditure of Ministry of Health, 171; as most important Colombian health program, 181; beneficiaries of, 172, 182; benefits generated from, 141; programs for, allotted by income group, 135; provision for, 96; services covered under, 182; tax liability of recipients of, 139, 140
Mazzola, U.: 28
Medical attention: quality of, 94
Medical-hospital care: allocation of expenditures on, 135, 137, 140; as expenditure of Ministry of Health, 171; beneficiaries of, 182-183
Mera, K.: United States federal income tax structure, 36
Mieszkowski, P.: general equilibrium model of tax incidence, 193, 195
Minister of Labor and Social Security, 109
Ministry of Agriculture: cooperation with Ministry of Health, 96
Ministry of Education: cooperation with Ministry of Health, 96
Ministry of Finance: 95; tax return data, 126
Ministry of Health, Chile: 75; expenditure of, 75
Ministry of Hygiene, 93
Ministry of Labor, 104
Ministry of Public Health: 93; 95; 96; 103; 109; 179-181; analysis of, 170; beneficiaries of services provided by, 181; campaign against endemic disease, 112; control over public health system, 114; determination of public sector vaccinated, 102; expenditures for medical-hospital care, 17, 103, 157; finances for vaccination campaign, 102-103; finances of, 118, 180; function of,

96; health expenditures of, 171; health services sponsored by, 114; incidence of benefits generated by, 132; incidence of expenditures of, 169; medical care division, 97; percentage of total national health expenditure, 115; policy document prepared by, 95; redistributive impact of health expenditures, 179; residual pattern, 180; rural sanitation provisions for, 100; sectional health service in, 115; SEM, 102; services, classified, 114; sponsor of health service to self employed rural workers, 110; urban sanitation projects, 102; use-of-services provided by, 189; utilization of medical care facilities of, 184; welfare institutions funded by, 104

Mishan, E.: 65; analysis of risks, 61, 63-64; compensating variation, 64; criticism of Hochman and Rodgers paper, 26; data gathered from survey, 64-65; evaluation of loss or saving of life, 57, 59-60; individual's response to change in risk, 60; willingness to pay, 85-86; willingness to pay for reduction in disease, 137

Money flow approach, 66

Money transfers: as government expenditure, 19; as source-of-income benefit, 48; measure of source-of-income benefit, 19

Morbidity, causes of, 112

Musgrave, R. and P.: analysis of budget incidence, 191; approach to public finance, 25; criticism of Hochman and Rodgers paper, 26-27; differential incidence, 78, 187; Distribution Branch, 194; distribution of income, 195; theoretical analysis of expenditure incidence, 193

Musgrave Commission, 184

National Cancer Institute, 103

National Coffee Fund: 130; 175

National Directorate of Hygiene, 93

National government: funds, 96; taxes levied by, 180

National Health Laboratory, 100

National Health Plan: health programs under, 181; preparation of, 104

National Health Service, Chile (SNS), 75

National Hospital Fund: establishment of, 95; role in coordination of rural health program, 112

National Institute for Municipal Development (INSFOPAL): function of, 102; water supply and sewage, 102

National Institute of Special Health Programs (INPES): benefits generated by, 101; provisions of, 182; rural sanitation, 100-101; Samper Martinez, 102

National Medical Service for Employees, Chile (SERMENA), 75

National Morbidity Census: demand for medical services, 103

National sales tax: allocation of, 131, 171

National Service for Eradication of Malaria: vaccination campaign of, 102

National tax revenue: coffee taxes and indirect taxes, 130

National Ten-Year Health Plan: 95, 114

National University: sponsor of health services to self-employed rural workers, 110

Net fiscal incidence: 179; defined, 17

Net fiscal residuum: 169; pattern of, 181

Netherlands: measure of elasticity of substitution among goods, 35

Net income gain, 22

Net income increases, 48

Net output approach, 58-59

Net Social Benefit: defined, 46-48

NNP, 58

Nonallowance for certain benefits, 86

Norway: measure of elasticity of substitution among goods, 35

Occupational Illness and Work Insurance: introduction of, 144; transfer of funds from, 187

Office of Planning of Ministry of Finance: income ceded to spouses, 128

Old Age Benefits, 144

Operational measure of redistribution, 187

Optimal supply of public services: 41-44, 82

PAHO. *See* Colombian ten-year health plan

Pareto: improvement, 59-60; optimal output, 41; optimum, 59

Pasilla: 175; payment of, 130

Paz de Rio: employer in iron works, 110

Personal income tax: allocation of, 126

Petty, Sir W.: economic value of human life, 57
Pigou, A.: rise and fall of imputed benefits, 34
Polibio Cordova, 119-120
Poor: effect of taxation on, 16
Potable Water: provision for, 94
Poverty: remedies for, 15
Powell, A. and Van Hoa, T.: 35; utility functions, 36
Primary distribution: Behrens and Smolensky, 78; defined, 78
Private benefits: allocation of, 139; generation of use-of-income benefits, 23
Private goods: defined, 22
Private health services received, 135
Private medical practice, 94
Progressive income tax, 15
Promotoras: 182; 183; 190-191
Public expenditures: beneficiaries of, 16; benefit measurements of, 67; consumption of, 23; costs incurred by government, 67-68; distributional impact of, 15; incidence of, by size classes of income, 16
Public finance: theory of, 18; neoclassicial approach to, 25
Public good: Samuelson, 40; household share, 49; optimal output for, 23
Public health: expenditures classified as, 171, 172; measurement of benefits, 57
Public health expenditures: beneficiaries by income class, 73; burden of payment for, 17; environmental improvement of, 73; hospital care, 68; net fiscal incidence of, 16; outlays for health centers, 73; public health, 68; sanitation, 68; shared costs for, 17; study of benefit incidence by income class, 57; use in income redistribution, 17
Public health services: marginal evaluation for, 84; received, 135; redistribution effects of, 93
Public interest approach: defined, 51
Public nonredistributive benefits: allocation and imputation of, 139, 171; defined, 24; generation of use-of-income benefits, 23
Public redistributive benefits: 52; allocation of, 139; generated by public services, 23; generation of use-of-income benefits, 23; willingness-to-pay, 24
Public services: beneficiaries of, 18; costs of, 44, 46; optimal provision of, 82, 187; purchase of as use-of-income benefit, 22

Quindio, sectional office of, 151

Ratio taxes paid by income group, 126
Redistribution: defined, 86-87; through government taxes, 78
Retention tax: 175; payment of, 130
Risk: compensation for community, 63; financial aspect of, 61, 63; involuntarily assumed, 61; psychic aspects of, 61, 63
Rural and Urban Sanitation: programs, 114
Rural Health Promoters: duties of, 113; training of, 112-113
Rural sanitation: beneficiaries of, 182; second most important program for poor, 182

Salary earners: measurement of net income gains, 21
Samper Martinez, 100
Samper Martinez Laboratory: preparation of vaccines, 102
Samuelson, P.: definition of public good, 40, 52
Sanitation: beneficiaries of expenditures on, 74; expenditures on, 69; 135; generation of benefits from, 140; programs, 97, rural, 171; urban, 171, 183
Santa Marta: sectional office of, 151, 187
Sectional branches: administrators of social security programs, 109
Sectional health services, 185
Sewage system: governmental provision of, 94
Short-run impact study: as limitation of cost-of-service method, 77, 84-85, 86; measure of incidence of public health expenditure, 88
Situado Fiscal de Poblacion: defined, 185
Situado Fiscal Territorial: defined, 185
Smith, A.: economic value of human life, 57
Snodgrass, D.: 135; incidence of consumption and investment expenditures, 82
Social and Preventative Medicine Department of the Medical Faculty of the National University, 112

Social opportunity cost: defined, 46
Social point of view approach: defined, 59; in evaluating loss or saving of life, 59
Social Security. *See* Colombian Social Security Institute (ICSS)
Social security payroll tax: bearers of, 146, 149
Society for the Construction of Hospital Establishments, Chile (SCEH), 75
Solidarity Fund: contributions to, 154; government transfers to, 144; ICSS utilization of, 187; of central government, 173; transfers from, 154; transfer of taxes to, 154; use of, 114
Source of income: 76, 196; benefits, 19, 24, 140, 189
Source of income benefits: attribution of, 171; defined, 48; estimates of, 118; forms of, 48; imputation of, 139; to government employees, 22; willingness-to-pay principle, 188
Special Health Projects Institute: policy document prepared by, 95
Special Research Division: function of, 100
Specific expenditure incidence, 21, 195
Stamp tax: 130; allocation of, 171
Status quo, 77, 85, 86, 88, 187, 188
Supply, elasticity of, 196
Superior Health Council: 96; creation of, 93

Tanzi, V., 15-16
Tariffs: distributional objectives of, 74
Taxation: equity of, 16; impact on economy, 151
Tax incidence: analysis of, 180
Taxpayer benefits: 52; generated by public services, 23
Tax return: 128, 129
Tax transfer system, 181
Thirsk, W.: theoretical analysis of expenditure incidence, 193
Total benefits, 82
Total benefits received: equation of, 77
Total tax revenue, 132
Transfers: *See* in-kind transfers; *see* money transfers

UNICEF: Colombian ten-year health plan, 95
United Fruit Company, Colombia, 110
United Kingdom: measure of elasticity of substitution among goods, 35
United States: 38; 39; 40; costs of sanitation in, 69; elasticity of marginal utility, income, 84; fiscal incidence study, 65; Gillespie's study, 67; hospital care, 69; measure of elasticity of substitution among goods, 35
Upper income groups: beneficiaries of public services, 18
Use of income: 140; 196; equal to cost, 118; generated by sanitary expenditures, 140; generation of, 173
Use of income benefits: 40; 49-50; 139; 189; Aaron and McGuire method, 49; allocation across income classes, 76; analogous to market value, 189; attribution of, 171; classification of, 139; defined, 48; education, 56; for beneficiaries of Washington, D.C. public health expenditures, 76; generated by public services, 21, 23; imputation of, 27, 137, 172; marginal evaluation for, 23; private, 23; 49; public nonredistributive benefits, 24, 49; public redistributive benefits, 24, 49
Utility function, 34, 189

Vaccination campaigns: 114; provision of by government, 94
Valle del Cauca, sectional office of, 151
Value in exchange: Aaron and McGuire, 49; estimates, 77
Venezuela: distribution of income, 124

Welfare gain or loss: generated by government expenditures, 18; of income class, 141
Welfare insurance plans, 94
WHO. *See* World Health Organization
Willingness-to-pay approach: 50; 77; 87; 180-182; Aaron and McGuire analysis, 40, 49; analysis of distribution of benefits, 144; as measurement of benefits of public services, 190; benefit incidence estimated on basis of, 118, 167; benefits estimated on basis of, 137, 184; Boskoff and Ziegler study, 38; by upper income groups, 18; determinants of, 39; distribution of benefits from health services estimated on basis

of, 167; estimated benefits from, 169, 180; expenditures allocated to income group using, 157; for allocation of medical benefits, 183; for estimation of benefit incidence pattern and net fiscal residual pattern, 181; for public redistributive benefits, 24; Greene, Neenan and Scott, 65, 66, 76, 83; imputation of use-of-income benefits, 28; in allocation of benefits generated by health expenditures, 132; incidence of health benefits based on, 140, 176, 178; incidence pattern indicated by, 141; index, 139; limitation of analysis, 77, 187-189; Mishan's approach likened to, 65; relation to income, 38-39; source-of-income benefits, 66; use in determining fiscal residual patterns, 141; used in health expenditure analysis, 171; used to determine ICSS benefits, 173; used to impute benefits of health care, 171; using allocation of benefits, 179; variation of, 181; Watson study, 38

World Bank, 15

World Health Organization (WHO), 95

Zero budget: 78-79; counterfactual, 86; primary distribution of, 87